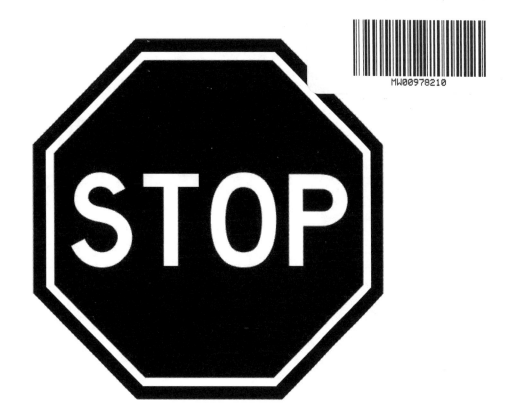

MW00978210

FREE Test Taking Tips DVD Offer

To help us better serve you, we have developed a Test Taking Tips DVD that we would like to give you for <u>FREE</u>. **This DVD covers world-class test taking tips that you can use to be even more successful when you are taking your test.**

All that we ask is that you email us your feedback about your study guide. Please let us know what you thought about it – whether that is good, bad or indifferent.

To get your **FREE Test Taking Tips DVD**, email <u>freedvd@studyguideteam.com</u> with "FREE Test Taking Tips DVD" in the subject line and the following information in the body of the email:

    a.   The title of your study guide.

    b.   Your product rating on a scale of 1-5, with 5 being the highest rating.

    c.   Your feedback about the study guide. What did you think of it?

    d.   Your full name and shipping address to send your free DVD.

If you have any questions or concerns, please don't hesitate to contact us at <u>freedvd@studyguideteam.com</u>.

Thanks again!

3 TEAS®
Practice Tests

Test of Essential Academic Skills
Version 5 Exam

Copyright 2016
By Exam Review Press

_____

All rights reserved

Copyright Notice
All rights reserved. No part of this book may be reproduced in any form by any electronic, mechanical, photocopying, recording, or otherwise, without written permission from the publisher.

*TEAS®, is a registered trademark of Assessment Technologies Institute®, which was not involved in the publication of, and does not endorse this product.

Table of Contents

Introduction

Thank you for your purchase of *3 TEAS Practice Tests: Exam Review Press*.

The TEAS is an important test, so it is essential that you adequately prepare for your test day. Be sure to set aside enough study time to be able to take each of the practice tests using only the amount of time that is specified. You are encouraged to minimize your external distractions in order to make the practice test conditions as similar to the real test conditions as possible.

Included are three complete TEAS practice tests. Each practice test is followed by detailed answer explanations.

The table below shows the amount of time and number of questions that are on each practice test. It is recommended that you use a timer when taking the test to properly simulate the test taking conditions.

Reading	Mathematics	Science	English and Language Usage	Total
48 items	34 items	54 items	34 items	170 items
58 minutes	51 minutes	66 minutes	34 minutes	209 minutes

DIRECTIONS: The questions you are about to take are multiple-choice with only one correct answer per question. Read each test item and mark your answer on the appropriate blank on the answer page that precedes each practice test.

When you have completed the practice test, you may check your answers with those on the answer key that follows the test.

Each practice test is followed by detailed answer explanations.

TEAS® Practice Test #1

Reading	Mathematics	Science		English and Language Usage
1. _____	1. _____	1. _____	49. _____	1. _____
2. _____	2. _____	2. _____	50. _____	2. _____
3. _____	3. _____	3. _____	51. _____	3. _____
4. _____	4. _____	4. _____	52. _____	4. _____
5. _____	5. _____	5. _____	53. _____	5. _____
6. _____	6. _____	6. _____	54. _____	6. _____
7. _____	7. _____	7. _____		7. _____
8. _____	8. _____	8. _____		8. _____
9. _____	9. _____	9. _____		9. _____
10. _____	10. _____	10. _____		10. _____
11. _____	11. _____	11. _____		11. _____
12. _____	12. _____	12. _____		12. _____
13. _____	13. _____	13. _____		13. _____
14. _____	14. _____	14. _____		14. _____
15. _____	15. _____	15. _____		15. _____
16. _____	16. _____	16. _____		16. _____
17. _____	17. _____	17. _____		17. _____
18. _____	18. _____	18. _____		18. _____
19. _____	19. _____	19. _____		19. _____
20. _____	20. _____	20. _____		20. _____
21. _____	21. _____	21. _____		21. _____
22. _____	22. _____	22. _____		22. _____
23. _____	23. _____	23. _____		23. _____
24. _____	24. _____	24. _____		24. _____
25. _____	25. _____	25. _____		25. _____
26. _____	26. _____	26. _____		26. _____
27. _____	27. _____	27. _____		27. _____
28. _____	28. _____	28. _____		28. _____
29. _____	29. _____	29. _____		29. _____
30. _____	30. _____	30. _____		30. _____
31. _____	31. _____	31. _____		31. _____
32. _____	32. _____	32. _____		32. _____
33. _____	33. _____	33. _____		33. _____
34. _____	34. _____	34. _____		34. _____
35. _____		35. _____		
36. _____		36. _____		
37. _____		37. _____		
38. _____		38. _____		
39. _____		39. _____		
40. _____		40. _____		
41. _____		41. _____		
42. _____		42. _____		
43. _____		43. _____		
44. _____		44. _____		
45. _____		45. _____		
46. _____		46. _____		
47. _____		47. _____		
48. _____		48. _____		

3 TEAS Practice Tests by Exam Review Press

Section 1. Reading

| Number of Questions: **48** |
| Time Limit: **58 Minutes** |

1. Adelaide attempted to <u>assuage</u> her guilt over the piece of cheesecake by limiting herself to salads the following day. Which of the following is the definition for the underlined word in the sentence above?
   a. increase
   b. support
   c. appease
   d. conceal

2. Hilaire's professor instructed him to improve the word choice in his papers. As the professor noted, Hilaire's ideas are good, but he relies too heavily on simple expressions when a more complex word would be appropriate. Which of the following resources will be most useful to Hilaire in this case?
   a. Roget's Thesaurus
   b. Oxford Latin Dictionary
   c. Encyclopedia Britannica
   d. Webster's Dictionary

The Dewey Decimal Classes
000 Computer science, information, and general works
100 Philosophy and psychology
200 Religion
300 Social sciences
400 Languages
500 Science and mathematics
600 Technical and applied science
700 Arts and recreation
800 Literature
900 History, geography, and biography

The next three questions are based on the above.

3. Lise is doing a research project on the various psychological theories that Sigmund Freud developed and on the modern response to those theories. She is not sure where to begin, so she consults the chart of Dewey Decimal Classes. To which section of the library should she go to begin looking for research material?
   a. 100
   b. 200
   c. 300
   d. 900

4. During her research, Lise discovers that Freud's theory of the Oedipal complex was based on ancient Greek mythology that was made famous by Sophocles' play *Oedipus Rex*. To which section of the library should she go if she is interested in reading the play?
   a. 300
   b. 400
   c. 800
   d. 900

5. Also during her research, Lise learns about Freud's Jewish background, and she decides to compare Freud's theories to traditional Judaism. To which section of the library should she go for more information on this subject?

    a. 100
    b. 200
    c. 800
    d. 900

---

6. Chapter 15: Roman Emperors in the First Century
- Tiberius, 14-37 AD
- Nero, 54-68 AD
- Domitian, 81-96 AD
- Hadrian, 117-138 AD

Analyze the headings above. Which of the following does not belong?

    a. Tiberius, 14-37 AD
    b. Nero, 54-68 AD
    c. Domitian, 81-96 AD
    d. Hadrian, 117-138 AD

---

7. Although his friends believed him to be enjoying a lavish lifestyle in the large family estate he had inherited, Enzo was in reality <u>impecunious</u>.

Which of the following is the definition for the underlined word in the sentence above?

    a. Penniless
    b. Unfortunate
    c. Emotional
    d. Commanding

---

8. Follow the numbered instructions to transform the starting word into a different word.

    1. Start with the word ESOTERIC
    2. Remove both instances of the letter E from the word
    3. Remove the letter I from the word
    4. Move the letter T from the middle of the word to the end of the word
    5. Remove the letter C from the word

What new word has been spelled?

    a. SECT
    b. SORT
    c. SORE
    d. TORE

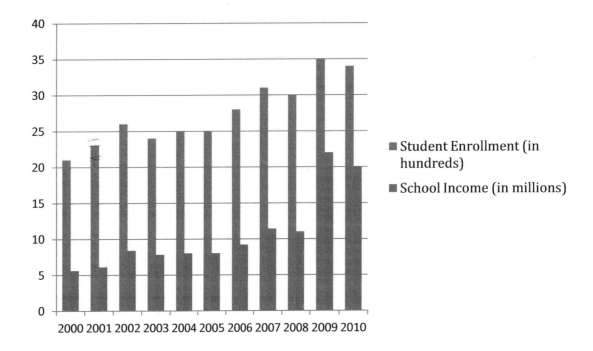

The next two questions are based on the above chart, which reflects the enrollment and the income for a small community college.

9. Based on the chart, approximately how many students attended the community college in the year 2001?
   a. 2100
   b. 2300
   c. 2500
   d. 2700

10. In order to offset costs, the college administration decided to increase enrollment costs. Reviewing the chart above, during which year is it most likely that the college raised the cost of enrollment?
   a. 2002
   b. 2007
   c. 2009
   d. 2010

11. The journalist, as part of his ongoing series of articles about the defendant accused of multiple murders, included a note that the defendant had written: "*No matter what they say I am not gilty [sic] of the crime.*" Which of the following does the bracketed expression "*sic*" indicate?
   a. An accidental misspelling in the sentence
   b. A grammatical error that the editor failed to catch
   c. An incorrect usage on the part of the original writer
   d. A point of emphasis that the journalist wants readers to see

The area known as the Bermuda Triangle has become such a part of popular culture that it can be difficult to separate fact from fiction. The interest first began when five Navy planes vanished in 1945, officially resulting from "causes or reasons unknown." The explanations about other accidents in the Triangle range from the scientific to the supernatural. Researchers have never been able to find anything truly mysterious about what happens in the Bermuda Triangle, if there even is a Bermuda Triangle. What is more, one of the biggest challenges in considering the phenomenon is deciding how much area actually represents the Bermuda Triangle. Most consider the Triangle to stretch from Miami out to Puerto Rico and to include the island of Bermuda. Others expand the area to include all of the Caribbean islands and to extend eastward as far as the Azores, which are closer to Europe than they are to North America.

The problem with having a larger Bermuda Triangle is that it increases the odds of accidents. There is near-constant travel, by ship and by plane, across the Atlantic, and accidents are expected to occur. In fact, the Bermuda Triangle happens to fall within one of the busiest navigational regions in the world, and the reality of greater activity creates the possibility for more to go wrong. Shipping records suggest that there is not a greater-than-average loss of vessels within the Bermuda Triangle, and many researchers have argued that the reputation of the Triangle makes any accident seem out of the ordinary. In fact, most accidents fall within the expected margin of error. The increase in ships from East Asia no doubt contributes to an increase in accidents. And as for the story of the Navy planes that disappeared within the Triangle, many researchers now conclude that it was the result of mistakes on the part of the pilots who were flying into storm clouds and simply got lost.

The next four questions are based on the passage above.

12. Which of the following describes this type of writing?
    a. Narrative
    b. Persuasive
    c. Expository
    d. Technical

13. Which of the following sentences is most representative of a summary sentence for this passage?
    a. The problem with having a larger Bermuda Triangle is that it increases the odds of accidents.
    b. The area that is called the Bermuda Triangle happens to fall within one of the busiest navigational regions in the world, and the reality of greater activity creates the possibility for more to go wrong.
    c. One of the biggest challenges in considering the phenomenon is deciding how much area actually represents the Bermuda Triangle.
    d. Researchers have never been able to find anything truly mysterious about what happens in the Bermuda Triangle, if there even is a Bermuda Triangle.

14. With which of the following statements would the author most likely agree?
    a. There is no real mystery about the Bermuda Triangle because most events have reasonable explanations.
    b. Researchers are wrong to expand the focus of the Triangle to the Azores, because this increases the likelihood of accidents.
    c. The official statement of "causes or reasons unknown" in the loss of the Navy planes was a deliberate concealment from the Navy.
    d. Reducing the legends about the mysteries of the Bermuda Triangle will help to reduce the number of reported accidents or shipping losses in that region.

15. Which of the following represents an opinion statement on the part of the author?
   a. The problem with having a larger Bermuda Triangle is that it increases the odds of accidents.
   b. The area known as the Bermuda Triangle has become such a part of popular culture that it can be difficult to sort through the myth and locate the truth.
   c. The increase in ships from East Asia no doubt contributes to an increase in accidents.
   d. Most consider the Triangle to stretch from Miami to Puerto Rico and include the island of Bermuda.

16. *But I don't like the beach*, Judith complained. *All that sand. It gets in between my toes, in my swimsuit, and in my hair and eyes.* Martin suggested an alternative. *Then, let's go to the park instead.* The use of italics in the text above indicates which of the following?
   a. Dialogue
   b. Emphasis
   c. Thoughts
   d. Anger

17. The guide words at the top of a dictionary page are *intrauterine* and *invest.* Which of the following words is an entry on this page?
   a. Intransigent
   b. Introspection
   c. Investiture
   d. Intone

18. The public eagerness to <u>lionize</u> the charming actor after his string of popular films kept his managers busy concealing his shady background and questionable activities.
Which of the following is the definition for the underlined word in the sentence above?
   a. Criticize
   b. Sympathize with
   c. Betray
   d. Glorify

19. Ninette has celiac disease, which means that she cannot eat any product containing gluten. Gluten is a protein present in many grains such as wheat, rye, and barley. Because of her health condition, Ninette has to be careful about what she eats to avoid having an allergic reaction. She will be attending an all-day industry event, and she requested the menu in advance.
   • Breakfast: Fresh coffee or tea, scrambled eggs, bacon or sausage
   • Lunch: Spinach salad (dressing available on the side), roasted chicken, steamed rice
   • Cocktail Hour: Various beverages, fruit and cheese plate
   • Dinner: Spaghetti and sauce, tossed salad, garlic bread

During which of these meals should Ninette be careful to bring her own food?
   a. Breakfast
   b. Lunch
   c. Cocktail Hour
   d. Dinner

20. Chapter 2: Shakespeare Before He Was Famous
- Family Background
- Childhood Experiences
- Education
- Dramatic Works
- Youthful Marriage to Anne Hathaway
- Move to London

Analyze the headings above. Which of the following does not belong?
a. Family Background
b. Education
c. Dramatic Works
d. Youthful Marriage to Anne Hathaway

21. *Letter to the Editor:*

I was disappointed by the August 12th article entitled *"How to Conserve Water."* While the author of the article, Neil Chambers, provided excellent tips, he overlooked the most obvious-- taking shorter showers. Mr. Chambers should consider the recent study by Dr. James Duncan on the subject, which examines the importance of shower length in reducing water use:

> While water conservation options vary, the most effective might also be one of the simplest. Consumers who take shorter showers can reduce their water usage significantly each year. The standard shower head allows releases more than two gallons of water per minute. By cutting each shower short by only five minutes, consumers can save over twelve gallons of water.

Water conservationists applaud the newspaper's efforts to direct readers toward opportunities to conserve, but journalists should put a little more effort into research before sending their work to publication.

Which of the following explains the reason for the indentation in the passage above?
a. A quote from another source
b. A conversation between two authorities on a subject
c. A quoted portion from a published article by the author of the letter
d. A disputed claim from the author of the newspaper article

22. With most of the evidence being circumstantial, the defense attorney was successful in his attempt to <u>exculpate</u> his client before the jury. Which of the following is the definition for the underlined word in the sentence above?
a. Dismiss
b. Clear
c. Condemn
d. Forgive

NAME	COMPOSITION (PER 100)	WORLD LITERATURE (PER 100)	TECHNICAL WRITING (PER 100)	LINGUISTICS (PER 100)
TEXTBOOK-MANIA	$4500	$5150	$6000	$6500
TEXTBOOK CENTRAL	$4350	$5200	$6100	$6550
BOOKSTORE SUPPLY	$4675	$5000	$5950	$6475
UNIVERSITY TEXTBOOKS	$4600	$5000	$6100	$6650

Note: Shipping is free for all schools that order 100 textbooks or more.

The next three questions are based on the above table.

23. A school needs to purchase 500 composition textbooks and 500 world literature textbooks. Which of the textbook suppliers can offer the lowest price?
    a. Textbook Mania
    b. Textbook Central
    c. Bookstore Supply
    d. University Textbooks

24. A school needs to purchase 1000 composition textbooks and 300 linguistics textbooks. Which of the textbook suppliers can offer the lowest price?
    a. Textbook Mania
    b. Textbook Central
    c. Bookstore Supply
    d. University Textbooks

25. A school needs to purchase 400 world literature textbooks and 200 technical writing textbooks. Which of the textbook suppliers can offer the lowest price?
    a. Textbook Mania
    b. Textbook Central
    c. Bookstore Supply
    d. University Textbooks

26. Given his fascination with all things nautical, Blaise could not pass up the opportunity to tour the reproduction 18th-century <u>bark</u> that was docked nearby. Based on the context of the passage above, which of the following is the definition of the underlined word?
    a. The outside surface of a tree
    b. A crisp order
    c. A piece of hard chocolate-coated candy
    d. A sailing vessel

27. A cruise brochure offers a variety of options for Mediterranean cruises. The brochure notes that the ships cruising the Mediterranean pull into the following cities:

- Venice, Italy
- Athens, Greece
- Barcelona, Spain
- Oslo, Norway
- Istanbul, Turkey

Which of these cities is out of place in the list above?
   a. Athens, Greece
   b. Barcelona, Spain
   c. Oslo, Norway
   d. Istanbul, Turkey

28. The same brochure provides customers with a list of cities in the United States from which the cruises depart:

- Baltimore, MD
- Boston, MA
- Charleston, SC
- Fort Lauderdale, FL
- _____
- Miami, FL

Consider the pattern in the list of cities above. Which of the following cities belongs in the blank?
   a. Tampa, FL
   b. Galveston, TX
   c. Norfolk, VA
   d. New York, NY

Starting Image

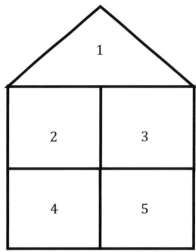

Start with the shape pictured above. Follow the directions to alter its appearance.
- Rotate section 1 90° clockwise and move it to the right side, against sections 3 and 5.
- Remove section 4.
- Move section 2 immediately above section 3.
- Swap section 2 and section 5.
- Remove section 5.
- Draw a circle around the shape, enclosing it completely.

29. Which of the following does the shape now look like?

a.

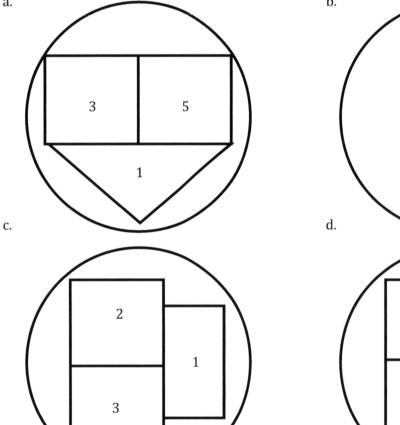

b.

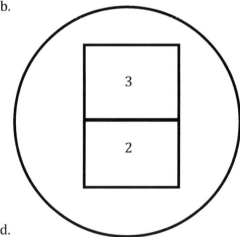

c.

d.

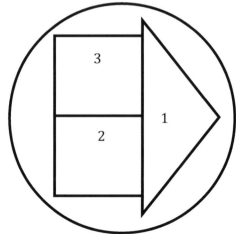

30. Anna is planning a trip to Bretagne, or Brittany, in the northwestern part of France. Since she knows very little about it, she is hoping to find the most up-to-date information with the widest variety of details about hiking trails, beaches, restaurants, and accommodations. Which of the following guides will be the best for her to review?
   a. *The Top Ten Places to Visit in Brittany*, published by a non-profit organization in Bretagne looking to draw tourism to the region (2010)
   b. *Getting to Know Nantes: Eating, Staying, and Sightseeing in Brittany's Largest City*, published by the French Ministry of Tourism (2009)
   c. *Hiking Through Bretagne: The Best Trails for Discovering Northwestern France*, published by a company that specializes in travel for those wanting to experience the outdoors (2008)
   d. *The Complete Guide to Brittany*, published by a travel book company that publishes guides for travel throughout Europe (2010)

Despite the aura of challenge that surrounds the making of haggis, Scotland's most famous dish takes some time but is really quite simple to prepare. Start with a sheep's stomach. Wash well, and soak for several hours. At the end of soaking, turn the stomach inside out. Boil one sheep's heart and one sheep's liver for about half an hour. Drain water and chop finely. Chop two or three onions. Toast approximately one cup of oatmeal, and then mix the chopped heart, liver, and onions with several spices: salt, pepper, cayenne, and nutmeg, seasoned to your preference. Add approximately one cup of the broth of your choice. Stuff the sheep's stomach with the mixture, and tie carefully with cooking twine. Make sure the stomach is well sealed. Then, add the stomach to a pot of boiling water, reduce to a simmer, and cook for about three hours. Have a needle ready to prick the stomach gently when it swells--it's better to avoid a haggis explosion!

31. Which of the following best describes the purpose of the passage above?
   a. Narrative
   b. Descriptive
   c. Persuasive
   d. Expository

---

207 HEATING AND AIR CONDITIONING
Furnace Cleaning
America's Heating Experts *204 Pine* (222) 850-1730
Everby Furnace *483 Maple*
        Duct Cleaning
        Free Estimates   (222) 850-3592
Good Ducts, Ltd. *983 Pine*   (222) 850-4829
Hebert Air *758 Sycamore*   (222) 850-2938
Furnace Installation
Everby Furnace *483 Maple*   (222) 850-3592
Fields Furnace Installation *399 Elm* (222) 850-5201
Young's Heating, Inc. *492 Elm*   (222) 850-2942
Furnace Parts and Supplies
Allen Heating & Air *394 Maple*   (222) 850-9605
US Best Furnace Supplies *603 Pine* (222) 850-3333
Wilkes Heating Parts *4930 Oak Alley* (222) 850-1940
Zimmer Furnace Parts *555 Cypress* (222) 850-2919
Furnace Repair
Ferris Furnace *706 Willow*
        Free estimates for all work (222) 850-4920
Perry Repairs *203 Sycamore*   (222) 850-3333
Thomas Refrigeration *849 Oak Alley*
        Call us 24 hours a day   (222) 850-9283
V&V Furnace Repair *492 Willow*
        Free estimates
        24-hour service   (222) 850-8694

Need Better Air?
Call Hebert!
Furnace Inspection
Duct Cleaning
Free Estimates For All Jobs
Call 222.850.2938

EVERBY
The Best in Furnaces
- Installation
- Cleaning
- Free Estimates
(222) 850-3592

Allen Heating
Expert Furnace Installation
Business Discounts
222-850-9605

Furnace on the Fritz?
Give FERRIS Furnace a Call!
-Discounts for First-Time Clients-
(222) 850-4920

Thomas Refrigeration
24/7 Furnace Emergencies
222-850-9283

The following two questions are based on the above image.

32. Edgar needs a new furnace, so he checks the telephone book for a local company that offers furnace installation services. He is also looking for a company that can provide cleaning after installation. Which of the following businesses should he call?
    a. Ferris Furnace
    b. Allen Heating & Air
    c. Everby Furnace
    d. Field's Furnace Installation

33. Pierre's furnace is not working properly, and he needs a repair service. Because it is already 11 PM, he is looking for a furnace repair business that offers 24-hour service. Since he does not know the extent of the damage, Pierre is also hoping for a free estimate. Which of the following businesses should he call?
    a. Ferris Furnace
    b. Perry Repairs
    c. Thomas Refrigeration
    d. V&V Furnace Repair

As little as three years before her birth, few would have thought that the child born Princess Alexandrina Victoria would eventually become Britain's longest reigning monarch, Queen Victoria. She was born in 1819, the only child of Edward, Duke of Kent who was the fourth son of King George III. Ahead of Edward were three brothers, two of whom became king but none of whom produced a legitimate, surviving heir. King George's eldest son, who was eventually crowned King George IV, secretly married a Catholic commoner, Maria Fitzherbert, in 1783. The marriage was never officially recognized, and in 1795, George was persuaded to marry a distant cousin, Caroline of Brunswick. The marriage was bitter, and the two had only one daughter, Princess Charlotte Augusta. She was popular in England where her eventual reign was welcomed, but in a tragic event that shocked the nation, the princess and her stillborn son died in childbirth in 1817.

Realizing the precarious position of the British throne, the remaining sons of King George III were motivated to marry and produce an heir. The first in line was Prince Frederick, the Duke of York. Frederick married Princess Frederica Charlotte of Prussia, but the two had no children. After Prince Frederick was Prince William, the Duke of Clarence. William married Princess Adelaide of Saxe-Meiningen, and they had two sickly daughters, neither of whom survived infancy. Finally, Prince Edward, the Duke of Kent, threw his hat into the ring with his marriage to Princess Victoria of Saxe-Coburg-Saalfeld. The Duke of Kent died less than a year after his daughter's birth, but the surviving Duchess of Kent was not unaware of the future possibilities for her daughter. She took every precaution to ensure that the young Princess Victoria was healthy and safe throughout her childhood.

Princess Victoria's uncle William succeeded his brother George IV to become King William IV. The new king recognized his niece as his future heir, but he did not necessarily trust her mother. As a result, he was determined to survive until Victoria's eighteenth birthday to ensure that she could rule in her own right without the regency of the Duchess of Kent. The king's fervent prayers were answered: he died June 20, 1837, less than one month after Victoria turned eighteen. Though young and inexperienced, the young queen recognized the importance of her position and determined to rule fairly and wisely. The improbable princess who became queen ruled for more than sixty-three years, and her reign is considered to be one of the most important in British history.

The next three questions are based on the above passage.

34. Which of the following is a logical conclusion that can be drawn from the information in the passage above?
    a. Victoria's long reign provided the opportunity for her to bring balance to England and right the wrongs that had occurred during the reigns of her uncle's.
    b. It was the death of Princess Charlotte Augusta that motivated the remaining princes to marry and start families.
    c. The Duke of Kent had hoped for a son but was delighted with his good fortune in producing the surviving heir that his brothers had failed to produce.
    d. King William IV was unreasonably suspicious of the Duchess of Kent's motivations, as she cared only for her daughter's well-being.

35. What is the author's likely purpose in writing this passage about Queen Victoria?
    a. To persuade the reader to appreciate the accomplishments of Queen Victoria, especially when placed against the failures of her forebears.
    b. To introduce the historical impact of the Victorian Era by introducing to readers the queen who gave that era its name.
    c. To explain how small events in history placed an unlikely princess in line to become the queen of England.
    d. To indicate the role that King George III's many sons played in changing the history of England.

36. Based on the context of the passage, the reader can infer that this information is likely to appear in which of the following types of works?
    a. A scholarly paper
    b. A mystery
    c. A fictional story
    d. A biography

In 1603, Queen Elizabeth I of England died. She had never married and had no heir, so the throne passed to a distant relative: James Stuart, the son of Elizabeth's cousin and one-time rival for the throne, Mary, Queen of Scots. James was crowned King James I of England. At the time, he was also King James VI of Scotland, and the combination of roles would create a spirit of conflict that haunted the two nations for generations to come.

The conflict developed as a result of rising tensions among the people within the nations, as well as between them. Scholars in the 21st century are far too hasty in dismissing the role of religion in political disputes, but religion undoubtedly played a role in the problems that faced England and Scotland. By the time of James Stuart's succession to the English throne, the English people had firmly embraced the teachings of Protestant theology. Similarly, the Scottish Lowlands was decisively Protestant. In the Scottish Highlands, however, the clans retained their Catholic faith. James acknowledged the Church of England and still sanctioned the largely Protestant translation of the Bible that still bears his name.

James's son King Charles I proved himself to be less committed to the Protestant Church of England. Charles married the Catholic Princess Henrietta Maria of France, and there were suspicions among the English and the Lowland Scots that Charles was quietly a Catholic. Charles's own political troubles extended beyond religion in this case, and he was beheaded in 1649. Eventually, his son King Charles II would be crowned, and this Charles is believed to have converted secretly to the Catholic Church. Charles II died without a legitimate heir, and his brother James ascended to the throne as King James II.

James was recognized to be a practicing Catholic, and his commitment to Catholicism would prove to be his downfall. James's wife Mary Beatrice lost a number of children during their infancy, and when she became pregnant again in 1687 the public became concerned. If James had a son, that son would undoubtedly be raised a Catholic, and the English people would not stand for this. Mary gave birth to a son, but the story quickly circulated that the royal child had died and the child named James's heir was a foundling smuggled in. James, his wife, and his infant son were forced to flee; and James's Protestant daughter Mary was crowned the queen.

In spite of a strong resemblance to the king, the young James was generally rejected among the English and the Lowland Scots, who referred to him as "the Pretender." But in the Highlands the Catholic princeling was welcomed. He inspired a group known as *Jacobites*, to reflect the Latin version of his name. His own son Charles, known affectionately as Bonnie Prince Charlie, would eventually raise an army and attempt to recapture what he believed to be his throne. The movement was soundly defeated at the Battle of Culloden in 1746, and England and Scotland have remained ostensibly Protestant ever since.

The next seven questions are based on this passage.

37. Which of the following sentences contains an opinion on the part of the author?
    a. James was recognized to be a practicing Catholic, and his commitment to Catholicism would prove to be his downfall.
    b. James' son King Charles I proved himself to be less committed to the Protestant Church of England.
    c. The movement was soundly defeated at the Battle of Culloden in 1746, and England and Scotland have remained ostensibly Protestant ever since.
    d. Scholars in the 21st century are far too hasty in dismissing the role of religion in political disputes, but religion undoubtedly played a role in the problems that faced England and Scotland.

38. Which of the following represents the best meaning of the word *foundling*, based on the context in the passage?
    a. Orphan
    b. Outlaw
    c. Charlatan
    d. Delinquent

39. Which of the following is a logical conclusion based on the information that is provided within the passage?
    a. Like Elizabeth I, Charles II never married and thus never had children.
    b. The English people were relieved each time that James II's wife Mary lost another child, as this prevented the chance of a Catholic monarch.
    c. Charles I's beheading had less to do with religion than with other political problems that England was facing.
    d. Unlike his son and grandsons, King James I had no Catholic leanings and was a faithful follower of the Protestant Church of England.

40. Based on the information that is provided within the passage, which of the following can be inferred about King James II's son?
    a. Considering his resemblance to King James II, the young James was very likely the legitimate child of the king and the queen.
    b. Given the queen's previous inability to produce a healthy child, the English and the Lowland Scots were right in suspecting the legitimacy of the prince.
    c. James "the Pretender" was not as popular among the Highland clans as his son Bonnie Prince Charlie.
    d. James was unable to acquire the resources needed to build the army and plan the invasion that his son succeeded in doing.

41. The use of the word *ostensibly* in the final paragraph suggests which of the following?
    a. Many of the monarchs of England and Scotland since 1746 have been secretly Catholic.
    b. The Catholic faith is unwelcome in England and Scotland, and Catholics have been persecuted over the centuries.
    c. The Highland clans of Scotland were required to give up their Catholic faith after the Battle of Culloden in 1746.
    d. While Catholics remain within England and Scotland, the two nations profess the Protestant Church of England as the primary church.

42. Which of the following best describes the organization of the information in the passage?
    a. Cause-effect
    b. Chronological sequence
    c. Problem-solution
    d. Comparison-contrast

43. Which of the following best describes the author's intent in the passage?
    a. To persuade
    b. To entertain
    c. To express feeling
    d. To inform

The instructor of a history class has just finished grading the essay exams from his students, and the results are not good. The essay exam was worth 70% of the final course score. The highest score in the class was a low B, and more than half of the class of 65 students failed the exam. In view of this, the instructor reconsiders his grading plan for the semester and sends out an email message to all students.

Dear Students:

The scores for the essay exam have been posted in the online course grade book. By now, many of you have probably seen your grade and are a little concerned. (And if you're not concerned, you should be--at least a bit!) At the beginning of the semester, I informed the class that I have a strict grading policy and that all scores will stand unquestioned. With each class comes a new challenge, however, and as any good instructor will tell you, sometimes the original plan has to change. As a result, I propose the following options for students to make up their score:

1) I will present the class with an extra credit project at the next course meeting. The extra credit project will be worth 150% of the point value of the essay exam that has just been completed. While I will not drop the essay exam score, I will give you more than enough of a chance to make up the difference and raise your overall score.

2) I will allow each student to develop his or her own extra credit project. This project may reflect the tenor of option number 1 (above) but will allow the student to create a project more in his or her own line of interest. Bear in mind, however, that this is more of a risk. The scoring for option number 2 will be more subjective to whether or not I feel that the project is a successful alternative to the essay exam. If it is, the student will be awarded up to 150% of the point value of the essay exam.

3) I will provide the class with the option of developing a group project. Students may form groups of 3 to 4 and put together an extra credit project that reflects a stronger response to the questions in the essay exam. This extra credit project will also be worth 150% of the point value of the essay exam. Note that each

student will receive an equal score for the project, so there is a risk in this as well. If you are part of a group in which you do most of the work, each member of the group will receive equal credit for it. The purpose of the group project is to allow students to work together and arrive at a stronger response than if each worked individually.

If you are interested in pursuing extra credit to make up for the essay exam, please choose <u>one</u> of the options above. No other extra credit opportunities will be provided for the course.

Good luck!

Dr. Edwards

The next three questions are based on the above passage.

44. Which of the following describes this type of writing?
    a. Technical
    b. Narrative
    c. Persuasive
    d. Expository

45. Which of the following best describes the instructor's purpose in writing this email to his students?
    a. To berate students for the poor scores that they made on the recent essay exam.
    b. To encourage students to continue working hard in spite of failure.
    c. To give students the opportunity to make up the bad score and avoid failing the course.
    d. To admit that the essay exam was likely too difficult for most students.

46. Which of the following offers the best summary for the instructor's motive in sending the email to the students?
    a. By now, many of you have probably seen your grade and are a little concerned. (And if you're not concerned, you should be--at least a bit!)
    b. With each class comes a new challenge, however, and as any good instructor will tell you, sometimes the original plan has to change.
    c. The purpose of the group project is to allow students to work together and arrive at a stronger response than if each worked individually.
    d. At the beginning of the semester, I informed the class that I have a strict grading policy and that all scores will stand unquestioned.

The following memo was posted to a company message board for all employees to review.

To all employees:

It has come to my attention that food items are disappearing from the refrigerator in the break room. Despite the fact that many of the items are unlabeled, they still belong to the individuals who brought them. Because of the food thefts, a number of employees have gone without lunch or have had to purchase a lunch after already bringing one for the day. This is both inconvenient and costly.

This is also unacceptable. Our company prides itself on hiring employees who respect others, and there is no excuse for taking what does not belong to you. Any employee caught taking an item out of the refrigerator that does not belong to him or her risks termination. (As a quick reminder, we encourage those who bring food items to label those items.) Demonstrate courtesy to your colleagues, and respect what is theirs.

In other words, if you didn't bring it, don't eat it.

Alicia Jones

Human Resources Manager

The next two questions are based on the above passage

47. Which of the following is the human resources manager's intent in the memo?
    a. To persuade
    b. To entertain
    c. To inform
    d. To express feelings

48. Which of the following explains the reason for the parenthetical note about employees labeling their food items?
    a. The labeling represents a kind of courtesy to the other employees to show which items belong to whom.
    b. The labeling ensures that the company will know whether or not an employee is removing his or her own item.
    c. The labeling represents a rule for employees who bring food, and the company can terminate employees that do not label food items.
    d. The labeling will enable the company to keep track of what is in the refrigerator and ensure that all employees are eating lunch.

Section 2. Mathematics

Number of Questions: **34**

Time Limit: **51 Minutes**

1. Which of the following is the percent equivalent of 0.0016?
    a. 16%
    b. 160%
    c. 1.6%
    d. 0.16%

2. Curtis is taking a road trip through Germany, where all distance signs are in metric. He passes a sign that states the city of Dusseldorf is 45 kilometers away. Approximately how far is this in miles?
    a. 42 miles
    b. 37 miles
    c. 28 miles
    d. 16 miles

3. Which of the following is the Roman numeral representation for the year 1768?
    a. MDCCLXVIII
    b. MMCXLVIII
    c. MDCCCXLV
    d. MDCCXLIII

4. It is 18 degrees Celsius at Essie's hotel in London. What is the approximate temperature in degrees Fahrenheit?
    a. 25
    b. 48
    c. 55
    d. 64

5. Pernell's last five consecutive scores on her chemistry exams were as follows: 81, 92, 87, 89, 94. What is the approximate average of her scores?
    a. 81
    b. 84
    c. 89
    d. 91

6. What is the *median* of Pernell's scores, as listed in the question above?
    a. 87
    b. 89
    c. 92
    d. 94

7. Gordon purchased a television when his local electronics store had a sale. The television was offered at 30% off its original price of $472. What was the sale price that Gordon paid?
    a. $141.60
    b. $225.70
    c. $305.30
    d. $330.40

8. $\frac{2}{3} \div \frac{4}{15} \times \frac{5}{8}$
Simplify the expression above. Which of the following is correct?
    a. $1\frac{9}{16}$
    b. $1\frac{1}{4}$
    c. $2\frac{1}{8}$
    d. 2

9. 0.0178 x 2.401
Simplify the expression above. Which of the following is correct?
    a. 2.0358414
    b. 0.0427378
    c. 0.2341695
    d. 0.3483240

10. Murray makes $1143.50 for each pay period, and the payments are deposited into his checking account twice a month. His monthly expenses currently include rent at $900 per month, utilities at $250 per month, car insurance at $45 per month, and the cost of food at $300 per month. Murray is trying to put away some money into a separate savings account each month, but he also wants to make sure he has at least $300 left over from his monthly expenses before putting any money into savings. Calculating all of Murray's monthly expenses, including the $300 he wants to keep in his checking account, how much money can he put into the savings account each month?
    a. $192
    b. $292
    c. $392
    d. $492

11. $4(2x - 6) = 10x - 6$
Solve for x above. Which of the following is correct?
    a. 5
    b. −7
    c. −9
    d. 10

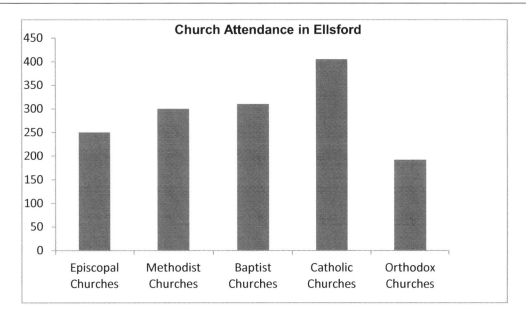

Church Attendance in Ellsford

12. The graph above shows the weekly church attendance among residents in the town of Ellsford, with the town having five different denominations: Episcopal, Methodist, Baptist, Catholic, and Orthodox. Approximately what percentage of church-goers in Ellsford attends Catholic churches?
   a. 23%
   b. 28%
   c. 36%
   d. 42%

13. Erma has her eye on two sweaters at her favorite clothing store, but she has been waiting for the store to offer a sale. This week, the store advertises that all clothing purchases, including sweaters, come with an incentive: 25% off a second item of equal or lesser value. One sweater is $50 and the other is $44. If Erma purchases the sweaters during the sale, what will she spend?
   a. $79
   b. $81
   c. $83
   d. $85

14. Sara plans to set up a booth at an industry fair. The cost for the booth is $500. Additionally, she is planning to give each person who visits the booth a pamphlet about her company and a key chain with the company's logo on it. Fair attendance is expected to be around 1500 people, but Sara expects that she will have only half that many people stop by the booth. As a result, she is only planning to bring pamphlets and key chains for 750 people. The cost of each pamphlet is $0.25 and the cost for each key chain is $0.75. What will Sara's overall cost be?
   a. $750
   b. $900
   c. $1000
   d. $1250

15. $4\frac{2}{3} \div 1\frac{1}{6}$

Simplify the expression above. Which of the following is correct?

    a. 2

    b. $3\frac{1}{3}$

    c. 4

    d. $4\frac{1}{2}$

16. 1.034 + 0.275 – 1.294

Simplify the expression above. Which of the following is correct?

    a. 0.015

    b. 0.15

    c. 1.5

    d. -0.15

17. $(2x + 4)(x - 6)$

Simplify the expression above. Which of the following is correct?

    a. $2x^2 + 8x - 24$

    b. $2x^2 + 8x + 24$

    c. $2x^2 - 8x + 24$

    d. $2x^2 - 8x - 24$

18. On the back of a video case, Digby notices that the listed date of production is MCMXCIV. What is this date in Arabic numerals?

    a. 1991

    b. 1994

    c. 1987

    d. 2003

19. If Stella's current weight is 56 kilograms, which of the following is her approximate weight in pounds. (Note: 1 kilogram is approximately equal to 2.2 pounds.)

    a. 123 pounds

    b. 110 pounds

    c. 156 pounds

    d. 137 pounds

20. Zander is paid $8.50 per hour at his full-time job. He typically works there from 8 AM to 5 PM each weekday, with a one-hour lunch break. The job offers no vacation benefits, so if Zander does not work, he does not get paid. Last week, he worked his full daily schedule of 8 hours each day, except for Wednesday when he left at 3:30 PM. Zander did take his lunch break that day. Which of the following is Zander's pay for the week?

    a. $318.50

    b. $327.25

    c. $335.75

    d. $340

21. $|2x - 7| = 3$
Solve the expression above for x. Which of the following is correct?
    a. $x = 4, 1$
    b. $x = 3, 0$
    c. $x = -2, 6$
    d. $x = 5, 2$

22. Between the years 2000 and 2010, the number of births in the town of Daneville increased from 1432 to 2219. Which of the following is the approximate percent of increase in the number of births during those ten years?
    a. 55%
    b. 36%
    c. 64%
    d. 42%

23. $\frac{1}{4} \times \frac{3}{5} \div 1\frac{1}{8}$
Simplify the expression above. Which of the following is correct?
    a. $\frac{8}{15}$
    b. $\frac{27}{160}$
    c. $\frac{2}{15}$
    d. $\frac{27}{40}$

24. While at the local ice skating rink, Cora went around the rink 27 times total. Cora slipped and fell 20 of the 27 times she skated around the rink. What approximate percentage of the times around the rink did Cora *not* slip and fall?
    a. 37%
    b. 74%
    c. 26%
    d. 15%

25. For her science project, Justine wants to develop a chart that shows the average monthly rainfall in her town. Which type of chart or graph is most appropriate?
    a. Circle graph
    b. Bar graph
    c. Pie chart
    d. Line graph

26. $3\frac{1}{6} - 1\frac{5}{6}$

Simplify the expression above. Which of the following is correct?

    a. $2\frac{1}{3}$

    b. $1\frac{1}{3}$

    c. $2\frac{1}{9}$

    d. $\frac{5}{6}$

27. Four more than a number, x, is 2 less than $\frac{1}{3}$ of another number, y.

Which of the following algebraic equations correctly represents the sentence above?

    a. $x + 4 = \frac{1}{3}y - 2$

    b. $4x = 2 - \frac{1}{3}y$

    c. $4 - x = 2 + \frac{1}{3}y$

    d. $x + 4 = 2 - \frac{1}{3}y$

28. $\frac{2xy^2 + 16x^2y - 20xy + 8}{4xy}$

Which of the following expressions is equivalent to the one listed above?

    a. $\frac{2}{y} + 4x - 2xy + 2$

    b. $2y + x^2y - 5 + \frac{xy}{2}$

    c. $\frac{y}{2} + 4x - 5 + \frac{2}{xy}$

    d. $\frac{x}{2} + 4xy - 16 + 2$

29. $4x - 6 \geq 2x + 4$

Solve the inequality above for x. Which of the following is correct?

    a. $x \geq 5$

    b. $x \geq 8$

    c. $x \leq 2$

    d. $x \geq 0$

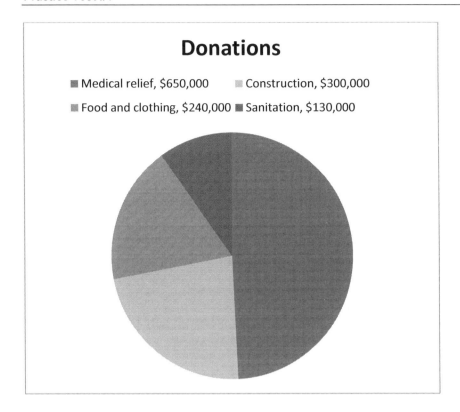

Donations

- Medical relief, $650,000
- Construction, $300,000
- Food and clothing, $240,000
- Sanitation, $130,000

30. After a hurricane struck a Pacific island, donations began flooding into a disaster relief organization. The organization provided the opportunity for donors to specify where they wanted the money to be used, and the organization provided five options. When the organization tallied the funds received, they allotted each to the designated need. Reviewing the chart above, what percentage of the funds was donated to support construction costs?
    a. 49%
    b. 23%
    c. 18%
    d. 10%

31. Margery is planning a vacation, and she has added up the cost. Her round-trip airfare will cost $572. Her hotel cost is $89 per night, and she will be staying at the hotel for five nights. She has allotted a total of $150 for sightseeing during her trip, and she expects to spend about $250 on meals. As she books the hotel, she is told that she will receive a discount of 10% per night off the price of $89 after the first night she stays there. Taking this discount into consideration, what is the amount that Margery expects to spend on her vacation?
    a. $1328.35
    b. $1373.50
    c. $1381.40
    d. $1417.60

32. $\dfrac{7}{3}, \dfrac{9}{2}, \dfrac{10}{9}, \dfrac{7}{8}$

Arrange the numbers above from least to greatest. Which of the following is correct?

   a. $\dfrac{10}{9}, \dfrac{7}{3}, \dfrac{9}{2}, \dfrac{7}{8}$

   b. $\dfrac{9}{2}, \dfrac{7}{3}, \dfrac{10}{9}, \dfrac{7}{8}$

   c. $\dfrac{7}{3}, \dfrac{9}{2}, \dfrac{10}{9}, \dfrac{7}{8}$

   d. $\dfrac{7}{8}, \dfrac{10}{9}, \dfrac{7}{3}, \dfrac{9}{2}$

33. Which of the following is the closest approximation of $\sqrt{30}$?

   a. 5.8

   b. 5.6

   c. 5.5

   d. 5.3

34. $7 + 4^2 - (5 + 6 \times 3) - 10 \times 2$

Simplify the expression above. Which of the following is correct?

   a. -23

   b. -20

   c. 23

   d. 20

| Section 3. Science | Number of Questions: **54** |
| | Time Limit: **66 Minutes** |

1. The first four steps of the scientific method are as follows:
    I. Identify the problem
    II. Ask questions
    III. Develop a hypothesis
    IV. Collect data and experiment on that data

Which of the following is the next step in the scientific method?
    a. Observe the data
    b. Analyze the results
    c. Measure the data
    d. Develop a conclusion

2. Which of the following best explains the relationship between science and mathematics?
    a. Mathematics offers different levels that science can use, such as geometry and trigonometry.
    b. Science provides the instruments that mathematicians need to complete calculations.
    c. Both help to improve the technology that is required for people to conduct their lives.
    d. Mathematics provides quantitative results that scientists can apply to theories.

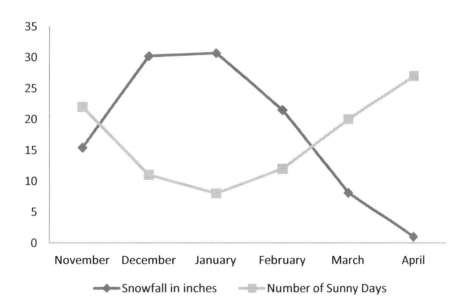

3. The chart above shows the average snowfall in inches for a town on Michigan's Upper Peninsula, during the months November through April. Which of the following can be concluded based on the information that is provided in the chart?
    a. April is not a good month to go skiing in the Upper Peninsula.
    b. Snowfall blocks the sunshine and reduces the number of sunny days.
    c. The fewest sunny days occur in the months with the heaviest snowfall.
    d. There is no connection between the amount of snowfall and the number of sunny days.

4. *Reading long books gives Benezet a headache.*
War and Peace is a long book.
Reading War and Peace will give Benezet a headache.
Which of the following correctly describes the conclusion that results from the three statements above?
   a. Inductive
   b. Irrational
   c. Relativistic
   d. Deductive

5. Every time Adelaide visits Ireland, it rains in Dublin. So far, Adelaide has visited Ireland seventeen times in the last three years, and she will visit Ireland again next week.
Which of the following is an *inductive* conclusion to the statements above?
   a. Adelaide should avoid Dublin during her visit.
   b. Adelaide should expect rain in Dublin next week.
   c. Adelaide's visits coincide with the rainy season in Ireland.
   d. Adelaide should put off her trip for a week to avoid the rain.

6. The two criteria for classifying epithelial tissue are *cell layers* and _____.
Which of the following completes the sentence above?
   a. Cell composition
   b. Cell absorption
   c. Cell shape
   d. Cell stratification

7. Which of the following types of connective tissue does *not* have its own (and thus limited) blood supply?
   a. Ligaments
   b. Adipose
   c. Bone
   d. Cartilage

8. Which of the following describes the number of organ systems that are in the human body?
   a. 12
   b. 15
   c. 9
   d. 11

9. Which element within the respiratory system is responsible for removing foreign matter from the lungs?
   a. Bronchial tubes
   b. Cilia
   c. Trachea
   d. Alveoli

10. Organized from high to low, the hierarchy of the human body's structure is as follows: organism, organ systems, organs, tissues. Which of the following comes next?
   a. Molecules
   b. Atoms
   c. Cells
   d. Muscle

Periodic Table

Note: the row labeled with * is the _Lanthanide Series_, and the row labeled with ^ is the _Actinide Series_.

The next six questions are based on the above chart.

11. On average, how many neutrons does one atom of bromine (Br) have?
   a. 35
   b. 44.90
   c. 45
   d. 79.90

12. On average, how many protons does one atom of zinc (Zn) have?
   a. 30
   b. 35
   c. 35.39
   d. 65.39

13. Which of the following has the highest ionization energy?
   a. Vanadium (V)
   b. Germanium (Ge)
   c. Potassium (K)
   d. Chromium (Cr)

14. Which of the following has the highest electronegativity?
    a. Gallium (Ga)
    b. Thallium (Tl)
    c. Boron (B)
    d. Aluminum (Al)

15. Which of the following would be least likely to chemically bond?
    a. Nitrogen (N)
    b. Sodium (Na)
    c. Calcium (Ca)
    d. Argon (Ar)

16. At 25 °C, there are two elements that exist as liquids: mercury and _____.
    a. Bromine (Br)
    b. Helium (He)
    c. Silicon (Si)
    d. Barium (Ba)

17. Which of the following describes one responsibility of the integumentary system?
    a. Distributing vital substances (such as nutrients) throughout the body
    b. Blocking pathogens that cause disease
    c. Sending leaked fluids from cardiovascular system back to the blood vessels
    d. Storing bodily hormones that influence gender traits

18. When are the *parasympathetic nerves* active within the nervous system?
    a. When an individual experiences a strong emotion, such as fear or excitement
    b. When an individual feels pain or heat
    c. When an individual is either talking or walking
    d. When an individual is either resting or eating

19. Which of the following best describes the relationship between the circulatory system and the integumentary system?
    a. Removal of excess heat from body
    b. Hormonal influence on blood pressure
    c. Regulation of blood's pressure and volume
    d. Development of blood cells within marrow

20. Once blood has been oxygenated, it travels through the pulmonary veins, through the left atrium, and then through the _____ before entering the left ventricle.
    a. Tricuspid valve
    b. Mitral valve
    c. Pulmonary arteries
    d. Aorta

21. *Fungi* are a part of which of the following domains?
   a. Archaea
   b. Archaebacteria
   c. Eubacteria
   d. Eukarya

22. Which of the following are the protein "messengers" that damaged cells release to within the immune system to signal the need for repair?
   a. Cytokines
   b. Perforins
   c. Leukocytes
   d. Interferons

23. The _____ of plant cells are larger than those of eukaryotic cells, because they contain water.
   a. Microtubules
   b. Vacuoles
   c. Flagella
   d. Nuclei

24. The three phases of interphase during mitosis are the following: G_1, G_2, and ____.
   a. V
   b. A
   c. S
   d. R

25. Which of the following is the number of possible *codons* within the code for genetic information?
   a. 16
   b. 32
   c. 64
   d. 128

26. Which of the following can cause mutations in human cells?
   a. Ultraviolet light
   b. Phosphate
   c. Proteins
   d. Nucleotides

27. Fill in the blanks below to complete the equation for photosynthesis:
CO_2 + _____ + Sunlight → _____ + Oxygen
   a. Glucose, Water
   b. Water, Chlorophyll
   c. Water, Glucose
   d. Chlorophyll, Glucose

28. Which of the following describes the purpose of a vaccine?
    a. Repairing damaged tissues that result from virus and/or cancer
    b. Signaling to the body the presence of a disease-causing pathogen
    c. Identifying the disease-causing pathogens that need to be destroyed
    d. Stimulating an infection to allow the body to produce its own antibodies

29. Which of the following cannot exist in RNA?
    a. Uracil
    b. Thymine
    c. Cytosine
    d. Guanine

30. Taking into account the answer the question above, which of the following exists in RNA, place of the substance above?
    a. Thymine
    b. Adenine
    c. Uracil
    d. Cytosine

31. The following four countries are listed in the order of their industrial development, from the greatest to the least amount of industrial development: Japan, Canada, Russia, and Namibia. Which of these countries can be expected to have the highest fertility rates?
    a. Namibia
    b. Canada
    c. Japan
    d. Russia

32. The development of characteristics that allow individuals within a species to survive and reproduce more effectively than others.
Which of the following terms best describes the theory that is defined above?
    a. Mutation
    b. Adaptation
    c. Allele combination
    d. Natural selection

33. In the development of genetic traits, one gene must match to one _____ for the traits to develop correctly.
    a. Codon
    b. Protein
    c. Amino acid
    d. Chromosome

34. Which of the following statements is true about genetic mutations?
    a. Most mutations result from disease.
    b. Mutations are never hereditary.
    c. Mutations due to harmful chemicals are rare.
    d. Most mutations are spontaneous.

35. Positively charged _____ are found *within* the nucleus of an atom, and negatively charged _____ are found *around* the nucleus.
    a. Protons, neutrons
    b. Electrons, neutrons
    c. Protons, electrons
    d. Electrons, protons

36. Which of the following best describes the careful ordering of molecules within solids that have a fixed shape?
    a. Physical bonding
    b. Polar molecules
    c. Metalloid structure
    d. Crystalline order

37. A *weak* bond in DNA often includes a(n) _____ atom.
    a. Oxygen
    b. Nitrogen
    c. Thymine
    d. Hydrogen

38. Which of the following describes the transport network that responsible for the transference of proteins throughout a cell?
    a. Golgi apparatus
    b. Endoplasmic reticulum
    c. Mitochondria
    d. Nucleolus

39. During the *anaphase* of mitosis, the _____, originally in pairs, separate from their daughters and move to the opposite ends (or poles) of the cell.
    a. Chromosomes
    b. Spindle fibers
    c. Centrioles
    d. Nuclear membranes

40. Which of the following is the *shortest* wavelength in the spectrum of electromagnetic waves?
    a. X-ray
    b. Visible
    c. Gamma
    d. Radio

41. The genetic code for DNA is composed of sequences of cytosine, thymine, guanine, and which of the following?
    a. Bromine
    b. Uracil
    c. Nitrogen
    d. Adenine

42. Which of the following offers the best definition of the *Law of Conservation of Energy*?
    a. Energy stores itself for future displacement and in the process preserves itself.
    b. Energy is displaced in motion and replaced in storage.
    c. Energy is never lost but is transferred from one form to another.
    d. Energy causes items in movement to remain thus unless stopped by another force.

43. A(n) _____ is the physical and visible expression of a genetic trait.
    a. Phenotype
    b. Allele
    c. Gamete
    d. Genotype

44. How many protons would a negatively charted isotope of N-12 have?
    a. 5
    b. 7
    c. 10
    d. 12

45. One or more _____ form during a reaction that results in atoms with unbalanced charges.
    a. Protons
    b. Neutrons
    c. Ions
    d. Electrons

46. A substance is considered *acidic* if it has a pH of less than which of the following?
    a. 12
    b. 9
    c. 7
    d. 4

47. Mutations occur as the result of mutagen-induced changes *or* which of the following?
    a. Duplication of a complete genome
    b. Errors during DNA replication
    c. Excision repair inspections of DNA
    d. Presence of germ cells within DNA

48. Which of the following describes the unit that is used to measure the distance between Earth and stars?
    a. Light-years
    b. Parsecs
    c. Nanometers
    d. Angstroms

49. Which of the following would be an example of *potential energy*?
    a. A ballet dancer performing stretches
    b A secretary typing at the computer
    c. A ball being thrown from one person to another
    d. A rubber band stretched to its fullest

50. Which of the following best describes one of the roles of RNA?
    a. Manufacturing the proteins needed for DNA
    b. Creating the bonds between the elements that compose DNA
    c. Sending messages about the correct sequence of proteins in DNA
    d. Forming the identifiable "*double helix*" shape of DNA

51. Which of the following do *catalysts* alter to control the rate of a chemical reaction?
    a. Substrate energy
    b. Activation energy
    c. Inhibitor energy
    d. Promoter energy

52. A metallic ion is considered a(n) _____, while a nonmetallic ion is considered a(n) _____.
    a. Metalloid, anion
    b. Anion, cation
    c. Covalent, cation
    d. Cation, anion

53. An unsaturated hydrocarbon with a double bond is considered a(n) _____, while an unsaturated hydrocarbon with a triple bond is considered a(n) _____.
    a. Alkane, alkyne
    b. Alkyne, alkene
    c. Alkene, alkane
    d. Alkene, alkyne

54. The Punnett square shown here indicates a cross between two parents, one with alleles BB and the other with alleles Bb. Select the correct entry for the upper right box in the Punnett square, which is indicated with the letter, x:

	B	B
B		x
b		

a. Bb
b. bB
c. BB
d. bb

Section 4. English and Language Usage	Number of Questions: **34**
	Time Limit: **34 Minutes**

1. Which of the following nouns represents the correct plural form of the word *syllabus*?
a. Syllabus
b. Syllaba
c. Syllabi
d. Syllabis

2. The Welsh kingdom of Gwynedd existed as an independent state from the early 5th century, when the Romans left Britain, until the late 13th century, when the king of England took control of Wales. Which of the following functions as an adjective in the sentence above?
    a. Independent
    b. Century
    c. Government
    d. Control

3. Hawaii's Big Island, the largest of the eight primary Hawaiian islands, _____ also the youngest of the islands. Which of the following is the correct verb for the subject of the sentence above?
    a. Are
    b. Is
    c. Was
    d. Were

4. Which of the following sentences shows the correct use of quotation marks?
    a. Grady asked Abe, 'Did you know that an earthquake and a tsunami hit Messina, Italy, in 1908?'
    b. Grady asked Abe, "Did you know that an earthquake and a tsunami hit Messina, Italy, in 1908"?
    c. Grady asked Abe, "Did you know that an earthquake and a tsunami hit Messina, Italy, in 1908?"
    d. Grady asked Abe, " 'Did you know that an earthquake and a tsunami hit Messina, Italy, in 1908'?"

5. Cody's dog lost _____ collar, so _____ mom made him rake the leaves to earn the money for a new one. Which of the following sets of words correctly fill in the blanks in the sentence above?
    a. Its; his
    b. It's; his
    c. His; its
    d. His; it's

6. Donald considered the job offer carefully, but he ultimately decided that the low salary was not
_____ given his previous experience. Which of the following is the correct completion of the
sentence above?
    A) exceptible
    B) acceptible
    C) acepptable
    D) acceptable

7. I'm usually good about keeping track of my keys. I lost them. I spent hours looking for them. I
found them in the freezer.

Which of the following options best combines the sentences above to show style and clarity?
    a. I lost my keys, even though I'm usually good about keeping track of them. I found them in the
       freezer and spent hours looking for them.
    b. I spent hours looking for my keys and found them in the freezer. I had lost them, even though
       I'm usually good about keeping track of them.
    c. I'm usually good about keeping track of my keys, but I lost them. After spending hours looking
       for them, I found them in the freezer.
    d. I'm usually good about keeping track of my keys, but I lost them in the freezer. I had to spend
       hours looking for them.

8. It was expected by the administration of Maplewood High School that classes would be canceled
because of snow. Which of the following best rewrites the sentences above so that the verbs are
active instead of passive?
    a. The administration of Maplewood High School expected to cancel classes because of snow.
    b. The snow caused the administration of Maplewood High School to expect that they would
       have to cancel classes.
    c. It was expected among the administration of Maplewood High School that the snow would
       cancel classes.
    d. It was the expectation of the Maplewood High School administration that the snow would
       cause classes to be canceled.

9. After living in Oak Ridge Missouri all her life, Cornelia was excited about her trip to Prague.

Which of the following best shows the correct punctuation of the city and the state within the
sentence above?
    a. After living in Oak Ridge, Missouri, all her life, Cornelia was excited about her trip to Prague.
    b. After living in Oak Ridge, Missouri all her life, Cornelia was excited about her trip to Prague.
    c. After living in Oak, Ridge, Missouri all her life, Cornelia was excited about her trip to Prague.
    d. After living in Oak Ridge Missouri all her life, Cornelia was excited about her trip to Prague.

10. Since each member had a different opinion on the issue, the council decided to rest until _____
could discuss the matter further at a later time. Which of the following pronoun(s) best complete(s)
the sentence above?
    a. It
    b. He and she
    c. They
    d. Each

11. The following words all end in the same suffix, *-ism*: polytheism, communism, nationalism. This suffix can apply a variety of meanings to words and suggest a range of possibilities, including a doctrine, a condition, a characteristic, or a state of being. Considering the meaning of these three words, how does the suffix *-ism* apply to all of them?
   a. Doctrine
   b. Condition
   c. Characteristic
   d. State of being

12. Which of the following sentences correctly uses quotes within quotes?
   a. Pastor Bernard read from the book of Genesis: 'And God said, "Let there be light." And there was light.'
   b. Pastor Bernard read from the book of Genesis: "And God said, 'Let there be light.' And there was light."
   c. Pastor Bernard read from the book of Genesis: " 'And God said, Let there be light. And there was light.' "
   d. Pastor Bernard read from the book of Genesis: "And God said, "Let there be light." And there was light."

13. Which of the following is an example of a correctly punctuated sentence?
   a. Beatrice is very intelligent, she just does not apply herself well enough in her classes to make good grades.
   b. Beatrice is very intelligent: she just does not apply herself well enough in her classes to make good grades.
   c. Beatrice is very intelligent she just does not apply herself well enough in her classes to make good grades
   d. Beatrice is very intelligent; she just does not apply herself well enough in her classes to make good grades.

14. Lynton was ready to make a commitment to buying a new car, but he was still unsure about which model would suit him best. Which of the following best removes the nominalization from the sentence above?
   a. Lynton was ready to make a commitment to a new car, but he was still unsure about which model would suit him best.
   b. Lynton was ready to make a commitment to buying a new car, but he was still unsure about the model that would suit him best.
   c. Lynton was ready to commit to buying a new car, but he was still unsure about which model would suit him best.
   d. Lynton was ready to make a commitment to buying a new car, but he was still unsure about which model was best.

15. Which of the following is a compound sentence?
    a. Tabitha and Simon started the day at the zoo and then went to the art museum for the rest of the afternoon.
    b. Tabitha and Simon started the day at the zoo, and then they went to the art museum for the rest of the afternoon.
    c. After starting the day at the zoo, Tabitha and Simon then went to the art museum for the rest of the afternoon.
d. Tabitha and Simon had a busy day, because they started at the zoo, and then they went to the art museum for the rest of the afternoon.

16. Which of the following follows the rules of capitalization?
    a. Dashiell visited his Cousin Elaine on Tuesday.
    b. Juniper sent a card to her Uncle Archibald who has been unwell.
    c. Flicka and her Mother spent the day setting up the rummage sale.
    d. Lowell and his twin Sister look alike but have very different personalities.

17. Historians tend to count Bede as the Father of English History, because he compiled extensive historical details about early England and wrote the *Ecclesiastical History of the English People*. Which of the following words does *not* function as a verb in the sentence above?
    a. tend
    b. count
    c. compiled
    d. wrote

18. We cannot allow the budget cuts to _____ the plans to improve education; the futures of _____ children are at stake. Which of the following sets of words correctly fill in the blanks in the sentence above?
    a. effect; your
    b. affect; you're
    c. effect; you're
    d. affect; your

19. The experience of being the survivor of a plane crash left an indelible impression on Johanna, and she suffered from nightmares for years afterwards.
Which of the following best explains the meaning of *indelible* in the sentence above?
    a. candid
    b. permanent
    c. inexpressible
    d. indirect

20. Which of the following sentences contains an incorrect use of capitalization?
    a. For Christmas, we are driving to the South to visit my grandmother in Mississippi.
    b. Last year, we went to East Texas to go camping in Piney Woods.
    c. Next month, we will visit my Aunt Darla who lives just East of us.
    d. When my sister-in-law Susan has her baby, I will take the train north to see her.

21. Which of the following nouns is in the correct plural form?
    a. phenomena
    b. mother-in-laws
    c. deers
    d. rooves

22. Which of the following sentences is grammatically correct?
    a. Krista was not sure who to hold responsible for the broken window.
    b. Krista was not sure whom was responsible for the broken window.
    c. Krista was not sure whom to hold responsible for the broken window.
    d. Krista was not sure on who she should place responsibility for the broken window.

23. Irish politician Constance Markiewicz was the first woman elected to the British House of Commons, but she never served in that capacity due to her activity in forming the Irish Republic. The word *capacity* functions as which of the following parts of speech in the sentence above?
    a. Verb
    b. Noun
    c. Adverb
    d. Pronoun

24. Which of the following sentences represents the best style and clarity of expression?
    a. Without adequate preparation, the test was likely to be a failure for Zara
    b. The test was likely to be a failure for Zara without adequate preparation
    c. Without adequate preparation, Zara expected to fail the test
    d. Zara expected to fail the test without adequate preparation

25. Valerie refused to buy the television, because she claimed that the price was exorbitant and _____. Which of the following phrases best completes the meaning of the sentence in the context of the word *exorbitant*?
    a. the quality too low for the cost
    b. within the expected price range of similar televisions
    c. much better than she had expected it to be
    d. far exceeding the cost of similar televisions

26. Which of the following sentences contains a correct example of subject-verb agreement?
    a. All of the board members are in agreement on the issue.
    b. Each of the students were concerned about the test scores for the final exam.
    c. Neither of the children are at home right now.
    d. Any of the brownie recipes are perfect for the bake sale.

27. Clemence and I went to the library together, and then _____ stopped to get some coffee. Which of the following phrases correctly fills in the blanks in the sentence above?
    a. her and I
    b. her and me
    c. she and I
    d. me and her

28. Burton sent the Christmas card to ____ and ____. Which of the following sets of words correctly fills in the blanks in the sentence above?
    a. her; me
    b. she; me
    c. her; I
    d. she; I

29. Which of the following is a simple sentence?
    a. Phillippa walked the dog, and Primula gave the dog a bath.
    b. Phillippa walked and bathed the dog, and Primula helped.
    c. Phillippa walked the dog, while Primula gave the dog a bath.
d. Phillippa and Primula walked the dog and gave the dog a bath.

30. After the natural disaster struck the county of Hillsborough in Florida, the president declared a state of emergency for that region and promised immediate aid. Which of the following words or phrases in the sentence above should be capitalized?
    a. county
    b. president
    c. state of emergency
    d. aid

31. After his first three-act drama received great critical acclaim, Erastus is on his way to becoming a respected and established _____ in the community. Which of the following correctly completes the sentence above?
    a. play wright
    b. play write
    c. playwright
    d. play-write

32. Which of the following sentences is most correct in terms of style, clarity, and punctuation?
    a. The possible side effects of the medication that the doctor had prescribed for her was a concern for Lucinda, and she continued to take the medication.
    b. The medication that the doctor prescribed had side effects concerning Lucinda who continued to take it.
    c. Lucinda was concerned about side effects from the medication that her doctor had prescribed, so she continued to take it.
    d. Although Lucinda was concerned about the possible side effects, she continued to take the medication that her doctor had prescribed for her.

33. The jury reentered the courtroom after reaching _____ decision. Which of the following correctly completes the sentence above?
    a. it's
    b. they're
    c. its
    d. their

34. Amber was quick to _____ Romy on the way that she had arranged the eclectic pieces of furniture to _____ one another.

Which of the following sets of words correctly fills in the blanks in the sentence above?
    a. compliment; complement
    b. compliment; compliment
    c. complement; compliment
    d. complement; complement

Answer Explanations

Reading Answer Explanations

1. C: To *assuage* is to lessen the effects of something, in this case Adelaide's guilt over eating the piece of cheesecake. The context of the sentence also suggests that she feels sorry for eating it and wants to compensate the following day.

2. A: If Hilaire's vocabulary needs a boost, he needs a thesaurus, which provides a range of synonyms (or antonyms) for words. A dictionary is useful for word meanings, but it will not necessarily assist Hilaire in improving the words he already has in his papers. A Latin dictionary makes little sense in this case, since Hilaire needs to find stronger words in English instead of studying word origins or applying a translation. The encyclopedia is also irrelevant, particularly since the professor already approves of Hilaire's work and is not asking him to research further.

3. A: To find information on Freud's psychological theories, Lise should go to class 100.

4. C: In this case, Lise needs to find a work of literature instead of a work of psychology, so she should consult the 800s.

5. B: To study Jewish traditions further, Lise should consult the 200s, which is devoted to books on religion.

6. D: The first century comprises the years leading up to 100 AD. That means that all first century emperors will have reigns before 100 AD. Hadrian's reign began in 117 AD, so he belongs in the second century instead of the first.

7. A: The sentence indicates a contrast between the appearance and the reality. Enzo's friends believe him to be wealthy, due to the large home that he inherited, but he is actually penniless.

8. B: The word SORT results from following all of the directions that are provided.

9. B: The enrollment in 2001 falls directly between 2000 and 2500, so 2300 is accurate. Note that the enrollment for 2000 falls much closer to 2000, so 2100 is a best estimate for that year.

10. C: The tuition appears to rise alongside the enrollment, until the year 2009 when it jumps significantly. Since the enrollment between 2008 and 2009 does not justify the immediate jump in income for the school, an increase in tuition costs makes sense.

11. C: The word "sic" is Latin for "as such" or "so." It is used to indicate an error on the part of the original author and is used most often when writers are quoting someone else. If the journalist includes the letter as written by the defendant, this is a natural way to show that the misspelling of "guilty" is the responsibility of the defendant and not a typographical error on the part of the journalist.

12. C: The passage is *expository* in the sense that it looks more closely into the mysteries of the Bermuda Triangle and *exposes* information about what researchers have studied and now believe.

13. D: This sentence is the best summary statement for the entire passage, because it wraps up clearly what the author is saying about the results of studies on the Bermuda Triangle.

14. A: Of all the sentences provided, this is the most likely one with which the author would agree. The passage suggests that most of the "mysteries" of the Bermuda Triangle can be explained in a reasonable way. The passage mentions that some expand the Triangle to the Azores, but this is a point of fact, and the author makes no mention of whether or not this is in error. The author quotes the Navy's response to the disappearance of the planes, but there is no reason to believe the author questions this response. The author raises questions about the many myths surrounding the Triangle, but at no point does the author connect these myths with what are described as accidents that fall "within the expected margin of error."

15. C: The inclusion of the statement about the ships from East Asia is an opinion statement, as the author provides no support or explanation. The other statements within the answer choices offer supporting evidence and explanatory material, making them acceptable for an expository composition.

16. A: In this case, the italics suggest a conversation or a dialogue that is occurring between Judith and Martin. While quotation marks are standard for dialogue, the use of italics here is consistent in representing the conversation effectively.

17. B: Only the word *introspection* can fall between *intrauterine* and *invest*. The words *intransigent* and *intone* come before, and the word *investiture* follows.

18. D: The context of the sentence suggests a positive response from the public, so the word *glorify* makes sense as a definition here. There is nothing about the public's response that suggests they criticize or betray him, and the actor's management working to keep information about him private would indicate that the public is not given the opportunity to sympathize with him.

19. D: The spaghetti and the garlic bread are definitely concerns for Ninette if she is unable to consume products with wheat in them. With all other meals, there appear to be gluten-free options that she can eat.

20. C: A discussion of Shakespeare's dramatic works has no place in a chapter that describes his life before he was famous. All other options make sense in a chapter about his formative years and his experiences prior to moving to London and achieving fame.

21. A: The indented portion of the passage indicates that the writer of the letter to the editor is quoting another source (identified as an article by Dr. James Duncan). For long quotes (longer than three lines), it is standard to indent. Shorter quotes (those shorter than three lines) are typically placed in quotation marks and included within the main text of the paragraph.

22. B: The context of the passage suggests that the defense attorney successfully *cleared* his client. To *dismiss* his client would make little sense here. To *condemn* his client would go against his job description, and to *forgive* is not his job–that is the job of the state after the jury reaches its decision.

23. B: This question and the two that follow require simple multiplication and addition. The school needs 500 of each type of textbook. Textbook Central's price for the entire transaction is $47,750 ($4350 and $5200 for each group of 100 textbooks that are purchased). The only textbook supplier with the potential for a competitive price is Textbook Mania, but that company's total price is $48,250. Bookstore Supply's total cost is $48,375. University Textbook's total cost is $48,000.

24. B: Once again, Textbook Central prevails. In this case, it is not even necessary to do the calculations. The cost for composition textbooks is $4350 (per 100) and for linguistics textbooks is $6550 (per 100). The lower cost for the composition textbooks–$150 less per 100 than the closest company in cost–outweighs the slight difference in cost for the linguistics textbooks.

25. C: This question does not require any math. Bookstore Supply has the lowest cost of the four for the technical writing textbooks, and it has a comparable cost to University Textbook for the world literature textbooks. The slight difference for the technical writing textbooks will make the overall cost lower than University Textbook's and thus give Bookstore Supply the competitive edge in cost.

26. D: The key words in question 26 are *nautical* and *docked*. This indicates some type of sailing vessel, which is provided in answer choice D.

27. C: It does not require extensive knowledge of geography to know that Oslo, Norway is nowhere near the Mediterranean Sea. Clearly, this city is out of place in the brochure.

28. B: A closer look at the list indicates that the cities are arranged alphabetically by the name of the city. This means that Galveston fits alphabetically between Fort Lauderdale and Miami.

29. D: Answer choice D is the only option that correctly follows the instructions in the question. Sections 4 and 5 are removed; section 1 is placed on the right sides along sections 3 and 2; and there is a circle drawn around the entire shape. Answer choice A places section 1 in the wrong location and fails to switch sections 2 and 5. Answer choice B incorrectly removes section 1 altogether. Answer choice C changes the shape of section 1 to a rectangle and reverses sections 2 and 3.

30. D: Anna is ultimately looking for a good all-around guidebook for the region. *The Top Ten Places to Visit in Brittany* might have some useful information, but it will not provide enough details about hiking trails, beaches, restaurants, and accommodations. *Getting to Know Nantes* limits the information to one city, and Anna's destination in Brittany is not identified. *Hiking Through Bretagne* limits the information to one activity. These three guidebooks might offer great supplemental information, but *The Complete Guide to Brittany* is the most likely to offer *all* of the information that Anna needs for her trip.

31. B: The passage offers details about a process, so it is descriptive in focus. Narrative passages tell a story. Persuasive passages attempt to persuade the reader to believe or agree with something. Expository passages *expose* an idea, theory, etc. and provide analysis. The passage provided simply tells the reader how to do something.

32. C: Everby Furnace is located under both Furnace Cleaning and Furnace Installation, so that is the best place for Edgar to start in looking for a company to do both tasks.

33. D: Only V&V Furnace Repair mentions 24-hour service and free estimates on the work. Thomas Refrigeration mentions "24-hour emergency service" specifically, but any company that offers 24-hour furnace repair service is offering it to assist clients with emergencies.

34. B: The passage does not state this outright, but the author indicates that the younger sons of King George III began considering the option of marrying and producing heirs *after* Princess Charlotte Augusta died. Since she was the heir-apparent, her death left the succession undetermined. The author mentions very little about any "wrongs" that Victoria's uncles committed, so this cannot be a logical conclusion. The passage says nothing about the Duke of Kent's preference for a male heir over a female. (In fact, it was likely that he was delighted to have any heir.) And the author does not provide enough detail about the relationship between the

Duchess of Kent and King William IV to infer logically that his suspicions were "unreasonable" or that the duchess cared only for her daughter's well-being.

35. C: The author actually notes in the last paragraph that Victoria was an "improbable princess who became queen" and the rest of the passage demonstrates how it was a series of small events that changed the course of British succession. The passage is largely factual, so it makes little sense as a persuasive argument. The author mentions the Victorian Era, but the passage is more about Queen Victoria's family background than it is about the era to which she gave her name. And the passage is more about how the events affected Victoria (and through her, England) than it is about the direct effect that George III's sons had on English history.

36. D: This passage is most likely to belong in some kind of biographical reference about Queen Victoria. A scholarly paper would include more analysis instead of just fact. The information in the passage does not fit the genre of mystery at all. And since the passage recounts history, it is not an obvious candidate for a fictional story.

37. D: All other sentences in the passage offer some support or explanation. Only the sentence in answer choice D indicates an unsupported opinion on the part of the author.

38. A: The passage indicates that it was believed the child died and that he was replaced by another child. Since it is unlikely a parent would willingly give up a child, even for such a purpose, the supposed substitution must have been an orphan. The act would have been illegal, but that does not make the child himself an outlaw (answer choice B). An unknowing infant can hardly be accused of being a charlatan (answer choice C), nor is there enough information in the passage to accuse the infant of being a delinquent (answer choice D). It is likely that, if such a fraud was perpetrated, the child was simply an orphan.

39. C: The author actually says, "Charles's own political troubles extended beyond religion in this case, and he was beheaded in 1649." This would indicate that religion was less involved in this situation than in other situations. There is not enough information to infer that Charles II never married; the passage only notes that he had no legitimate children. (In fact, he had more than ten illegitimate children by his mistresses.) And while the chance of a Catholic king frightened many in England, it is reaching beyond logical inference to assume that people were relieved when the royal children died. Finally, the author does not provide enough detail for the reader to assume that James I had *no* Catholic leanings. The author only says that James recognized the importance of committing to the Church of England.

40. A: The author notes, "In spite of a strong resemblance to the king, the young James was generally rejected among the English and the Lowland Scots, who referred to him as "the Pretender." This indicates that there *was* a resemblance, and this increases the likelihood that the child was, in fact, that of James and Mary Beatrice. Answer choice B is too much of an opinion statement that does not have enough support in the passage. The passage essentially refutes answer choice C by pointing out that James "the Pretender" was welcomed in the Highlands. And there is little in the passage to suggest that James was unable to raise an army and mount an attack.

41. D: The context of the passage would suggest that Catholicism is not necessarily absent in England and Scotland but that the Church of England is accepted as primary. The word *ostensibly* means *evidently* or *on the surface*, but this alone is not enough to suggest that many monarchs have secretly been Catholic. The passage offers no indication that Catholics remain unwelcome; and while persecution against Catholics is a historical fact, the passage offers no discussion about it. Additionally, there is not enough information in the passage to arrive at the conclusion that the Highland clans were required to give up their Catholic faith. It is a possibility, but it cannot be concluded by the use of the word *ostensibly*.

42. B: The passage is composed in a chronological sequence with each king introduced in order of reign.

43. D: The passage is largely informative in focus, and the author provides extensive detail about this period in English and Scottish history. There is little in the passage to suggest persuasion, and the tone of the passage has no indication of a desire to entertain. Additionally, the passage is historical, so the author avoids expressing feelings and instead focuses on factual information (with the exception of the one opinion statement).

44. A: Technical passages focus on presenting specific information and with a tone of formality. Narrative writing focuses on telling a story, and the passage offers no indication of this. Persuasive writing attempts to persuade the reader to agree with a certain position; the instructor offers the students information but leaves the decision up to each student. Expository passages reveal analytical information to the reader. The instructor is more focused on providing the students with information than with offering the students analytical details. (The analysis, it appears, will be up to the students if they choose to complete an extra credit project.)

45. C: Answer choice C fits the tone of the passage best. The instructor is simply offering students the chance to make up the exam score (which is worth 70% of their grade) and thus avoid failing the course. The instructor does not berate students at any point, nor does the instructor admit that the exam was too difficult. Additionally, the instructor offers encouragement to the students should they choose to complete an extra credit project, but that is not the primary purpose of this email.

46. B: This question asks for the best summary of the instructor's motive. In the opening paragraph, the instructor notes that his original grading plan has to change to reflect the exam scores. Because they were low, he now wants to give students a chance to make up that score. Answer choice B thus summarizes his motive effectively. The instructor introduces his email with the notes about the scores being posted, but, given the information that is provided in the message, this is not the sole motive for his writing. Answer choice A limits the motive to the details about the group project, and the instructor provides three options. Answer choice D overlooks the instructor's further note about how the grading policy sometimes has to bend to reflect circumstances.

47. C: The human resources manager is informing employees about the company's new policy regarding food items in the refrigerator and the consequences for breaking that policy. There is no overt persuasion in the passage–beyond the standard persuasion of telling people the rules and expecting them to follow those rules or face the consequences. (As a persuasive passage focuses on convincing someone to agree with or believe something, persuasion does not apply to this passage.) The memo has no tone of entertainment or the expression of feelings; it is simply informing employees of a new policy.

48. B: There is no mistake in the location of the parenthetical note. It directly follows the statement about possible termination for employees who take food items that do not belong to them. This indicates that the labeling will help the company recognize that employees are removing their own food items from the refrigerator. The human resources manager mentions the importance of respect or courtesy, but this is not the best explanation for the parenthetical note. There is no suggestion of termination for employees that do not label their food; the memo notes only that the company encourages labeling. The memo offers no suggestion that the company is interested in labeling beyond employees being able to eat their own food. There is no reason to believe that the company is trying to ensure that employees actually eat a lunch.

Mathematics Answer Explanations

1. D: To derive a percentage from a decimal, multiply by 100: 0.0016(100) = 0.16%.

2. C: One kilometer is about 0.62 miles, so 45(0.62) is 27.9, or approximately 28 miles.

3. A: In Roman numerals, M is 1000, D is 500, C is 100, L is 50, X is 10, V is 5, and I is 1. For the year 1768, the Roman numeral MDCCLXVIII is correct – representing 1000 + 500 + 200 + 50 + 10 + 5 + 3. MMCXLVIII is 2148 (still yet to be achieved) MDCCCXLV is 1845, and MDCCXLIII is 1743.

4. D: To convert from Celsius to Fahrenheit, start by multiplying by 9 and then dividing by 5. Add 32 to the quotient, and the conversion is complete. For question 4:

$$18(9) = 162$$

162/5 = 32.4

32.4 + 32 = 64.4, or approximately 64

5. C: To find the average of Pernell's scores, add them up and then divide by the number of scores (5 in this case). In other words,

$$81 + 92 + 87 + 89 + 94 = 443$$
$$443/5 = 88.6, \text{ or approximately } 89$$

6. B: To find the median, list the series of numbers from least to greatest. The middle number represents the median--in this case 81, 87, 89, 92, 94. The number 89 is in the middle, so it is the median.

7. D: The television is 30% off its original price of $472. Therefore, 30% of 472 is 141.60, and 141.60 subtracted from 472 is 330.40. Thus, Gordon pays $330.40 for the television.

8. A: To simplify, proceed in the order of the operations: $\frac{2}{3} \div \frac{4}{15}$ is $\frac{2}{3} \times \frac{15}{4}$, or $\frac{5}{2}$. Next, multiply $\frac{5}{2}$ by $\frac{5}{28}$. The result is $\frac{25}{16}$, or $1\frac{9}{16}$.

9. B: Question 9 is a simple matter of multiplication. The product is 0.0427378.

10. D: Start by multiplying Murray's payment by 2, since he receives this twice a month: $2287. Subtract all of his expenses, including the $300 he plans to keep in his checking account. The amount of $492 is left over, and this is what Murray can plan to put in his savings account each month, as long as his expenses remain the same.

11. C: Multiplying the equation results in the following:

$$8x - 24 = 10x - 6$$
$$-18 = 2x$$
$$x = -\frac{18}{2}, or - 9$$

12. B: Adding up the number of church-goers in Ellsford results in about 1450 residents who attend a church in the town each week. There are approximately 400 people in Ellsford who attend a Catholic church each week. This number represents about 28% of the 1450 church-goers in the town.

13. C: Erma's sale discount will be applied to the less expensive sweater, so she will receive the $44 sweater for 25% off. This amounts to a discount of $11, so the cost of the sweater will be $33. Added to the cost of the $50 sweater, which is not discounted, Erma's total is $83.

14. D: The combined cost of the pamphlets (750 at $0.25 each) and the key chains (750 at $0.75 each) is $750. With the cost of the booth ($500), Erma will pay a total of $1250.

15. C: Turn both expressions into fractions, and then multiply the first by the reverse of the second:
$$\frac{14}{3} \div \frac{7}{6}$$
$$\frac{14}{3} \times \frac{6}{7}$$
The result is the whole number 4.

16. A: Start by adding the first two expressions, and then subtract 1.294 from the sum:
$$1.034 + 0.275 = 1.309$$
$$1.309 - 1.294$$
The result is 0.015.

17. D: Multiply in the required order, and then add: $(2x)(x) + (2x)(-6) + (4)(x) + (4)(-6)$. The result is $2x^2 - 8x - 24$.

18. B: Recall that in Roman numerals, M is 1000, D is 500, C is 100, L is 50, X is 10, V is 5, and I is 1. As a result, the year MCMXCIV is 1994. (Note that the I before the V indicates that the I is subtracted from V: 5 – 1, or 4. In the same way, the C before the M also indicates a subtraction, in this case 100 from 1000, or 900.)

19. A: To find the correct answer, simply multiply 56 by 2.2. The result is 123.2, or approximately 123. This is Stella's weight in pounds.

20. B: To find the correct answer, start by adding up what Zander makes for the four full days he works: $8.50 per hours for 32 hours (four full 8-hour days). The result is $272. Then, add up what Zander makes on Wednesday when he leaves at 3:30 but still takes his standard one-hour lunch break. By leaving at 3:30, Zander only works 6.5 hours that day. At $8.50 per hour, this is $55.25 for the day. Added to $272, the result is $327.25.

21. D: Absolute value is determined by the distance between a number and 0 when plotted on a number line. For instance, the absolute value of –5 is 5. To solve the equation in question 21 for x requires the following:
$$|2x - 7| = 3$$
$$2x - 7 = 3, or\ 2x - 7 = -3$$
$$2x - 7 = 3$$
$$2x = 10, so\ x = 5$$
$$OR$$
$$2x = 4, so\ x = 2$$
The two possible solutions for the absolute value of the equation are 5 and 2.

22. A: Begin by subtracting 1432 from 2219. The result is 787. Then, divide 787 by 1432 to find the percent of increase: 0.549, or 54.9%. Rounded up, this is approximately a 55% increase in births between 2000 and 2010.

23. C: Solve the equation in the order of operations: $\frac{1}{4} \times \frac{3}{5}$, or $\frac{3}{20}$. Follow this up with division, which requires a reversal of the fraction: $\frac{3}{20} \div \frac{9}{8}$, or $\frac{3}{20} \times \frac{8}{9}$. The result is $\frac{2}{15}$.

24. C: Cora did *not* fall 7 out of 27 times. To find the solution, simply divide 7 by 27 to arrive at 0.259, or 25.9%. Rounded up, this is approximately 26%.

25. D: Justine's graph will be charting the amount of rainfall for each month. Line graph indicate change that occurs over a specified period of time, so this is the best type of graph for Justine to use.

26. B: Since the denominator is the same for both fractions, this is simple subtraction. Start by turning each expression into a fraction: $\frac{19}{6} - \frac{11}{6}$. The result is $\frac{8}{6}$, or $1\frac{2}{6} = 1\frac{1}{3}$.

27. A: The expression "Four more than a number, x" can be interpreted as $x + 4$. This is equal to "2 less than $\frac{1}{3}$ of another number, y," or $\frac{1}{3}y - 2$.

28. C: To solve the equation, start by separating each element:

$$\frac{2xy^2 + 16x^2y - 20xy + 8}{4xy}$$

$$\frac{2xy^2}{4xy}, \text{ or } \frac{y}{2}$$

$$\frac{16x^2y}{4xy}, \text{ or } 4x$$

$$-\frac{20xy}{4xy}, \text{ or } -5$$

$$\frac{8}{4xy}, \text{ or } \frac{2}{xy}$$

Combine: $\frac{y}{2} + 4x - 5 + \frac{2}{xy}$.

29. A: To solve, move the terms with x to the same side of the equation and the whole numbers to the other:

$$4x - 6 \geq 2x + 4$$
$$2x \geq 10$$
$$x \geq 5$$

You can test this answer by filling in a number greater than 5 to see if the inequality still holds. For instance with the number 7:

$$4(7) - 6 \geq 2(7) + 4$$

The number 22 (or $28 - 6$) is greater than (though obviously not equal to) 18 (or $14 + 4$), so the inequality works. The only time when the two sides are equal is when $x = 5$.
Note that answer choice B contains a number greater than 5 that also works to make the inequality correct (when the left side of the equation is greater than the right side). The number 8 works only for "greater than," however, and does not solve for "equal to," so answer choice B cannot be the correct answer.

30. B: Start by locating the section of the pie chart that represents construction. It looks close to a quarter of the pie chart, which means that it is probably 23%, but you can verify by adding up the numbers. The total donation amount is about $1.3 million and the amount given for construction is $0.3 million. 0.3/1.3 = 0.23 = 23%.

31. C: Start by adding up the costs of the trip, excluding the hotel cost: $572 + $150 + $250, or $972. Then, calculate what Margery will spend on the hotel. The first of her five nights at the hotel will cost her $89. For each of the other four nights, she will get a discount of 10% per night, or $8.90. This discount of $8.90 multiplied by the four nights is $35.60. The total she would have spent on the five nights without the discount is $445. With the discount, the amount goes down to $409.40. Add this amount to the $972 for a grand total of $1381.40.

32. D: Turn the fractions into mixed numbers to see the amounts more clearly. The result is that $\frac{7}{8}$ is smaller than $\frac{10}{9}$, or $1\frac{1}{9}$, which is smaller than $\frac{7}{3}$, or $2\frac{1}{3}$, which is smaller than $\frac{9}{2}$, or $4\frac{1}{2}$.

33. C: The square root of 25 is 5, and the square root of 36 is 6. The correct answer to the square root of 30 will have to be closely to the mid-point between 5 and 6. As a result, 5.5 is a good place to start testing, and it proves to be correct: $\sqrt{30} = 5.477$. This is approximately 5.5. (In exact terms, 5.5^2 is 30.25, but as this question only asks for the approximation, the answer of 5.5 is correct.) In comparison, 5.3^2 is 28.09; 5.6^2 is 31.36; 5.8^2 is 33.64. None of these is close enough to 30 to be correct.

34. B: Start by calculating the amount in parenthesis, completing the multiplication first: $5 + 6 \times 3$, which is $5 + 18$ or 23. Then calculate the product at the end: 10×2, or 20. Calculate the expression 4^2, for a result of 16, and complete the equation:

$$7 + 16 - 23 - 20$$
$$23 - 23 - 20$$
$$0 - 20, or - 20$$

Science Answer Explanations

1. B: There are six steps in the scientific process, the fifth of which is "Analyze the results" (the results of the experiments that were conducted in step four). The results of step four must be analyzed before reaching the final step, "Develop a conclusion."

2. D: Science and mathematics work together with mathematics offering the quantitative results that scientists can use to apply to their theories and thus prove whether or not they are correct.

3. C: The chart shows two specific changes: snowfall levels from November to April and sunny days from November to April. Based on the chart alone, the only information that can be determined is that the fewest sunny days coincide with the months that have the heaviest snowfall. Anything further reaches beyond the immediate facts of the chart and moves into the territory of requiring other facts. As for answer choice D, it uses the word "relationship," which is not required in the question. The question only asks for what can be concluded.

4. D: Deductive reasoning moves from the general to the specific. In this case, the general statement is that Benezet gets a headache from reading long books. The syllogism moves from the general to the specific by noting that *War and Peace* is a long book, therefore Benezet will likely get a headache from reading it.

5. B: Inductive reasoning moves from the specific to the general. In this case, the specific statement is that there is rain in Dublin every time Adelaide visits Ireland. The syllogism in this case moves from the specific to the general by then noting that Adelaide has visited Ireland 17 times in the last 3 years and that she will visit again next week. This is significant, because it raises the likelihood of rain. There is no guarantee of course, but the question merely asks for the inductive conclusion. To conclude the syllogism inductively, the best answer choice notes that Adelaide should expect rain in Dublin next week. All other answer choices move beyond the immediate syllogism and infer other information. (For instance, the first statement does not note that Adelaide actually visits Dublin but rather that she visits Ireland. It can rain in Dublin without Adelaide being there.) It is also possible to infer that Adelaide visits Ireland during the rainy season, but that is not a part of the original statement and therefore not possible as an inductive conclusion to the syllogism.

6. C: *Cell layers* and *cell shape* are the criteria for classifying epithelial tissue.

7. A: Ligaments do not have their own blood supply. As a result, ligament injuries tend to take longer to heal because they have a limited blood supply.

8. D: There are 11 organ systems in the human body: circulatory, digestive, endocrine, integumentary, lymphatic, muscular, nervous, reproductive, respiratory, skeletal, and urinary.

9. B: The cilia are the tiny hairs in the respiratory system that are responsible for removing foreign matter from the lungs. The cilia are located within the bronchial tubes, but it is the cilia that have the responsibility for removing inappropriate materials before they enter the lungs.

10. C: Cells come after tissues and are followed by molecules and then atoms at the very bottom of the hierarchy. Muscles are types of tissues, so muscles do not have a separate place in the hierarchy but instead fall within the types of tissues.

11. B: To determine the average number of neutrons in one atom of an element, subtract the atomic mass from the atomic number. For Bromine (Br), subtract its atomic number (35) from its atomic mass (79.9) to acquire the average number of neutrons, 44.9.

12. A: The number of protons is the same as the element's atomic periodic number: in this case, 30 for Zinc (Zn).

13. B: Ionization energy increases across a period (or row), from left to right. In the period containing the four elements listed in question 13, germanium (Ge) is the furthest to the right and thus has the highest ionization energy, also known as ionization potential.

14. C: Electronegativity increases in a group (or column) as the atomic number decreases–or put another way, the lower the atomic number, then the higher the electronegativity. Among the four elements listed in question 14, Boron (B) has the lowest atomic number (5) and thus the highest electronegativity.

15. D: As one of the noble gases, argon (Ar) is neutral and thus has no electrons for chemical bonding. As a result, it as well as the other noble gases in the period can resist chemical bonding.

16. A: Mercury and bromine are the only elements that are recognized as liquids in their natural state.

17. B: The integumentary system includes skin, hair, and mucous, and all are responsible–in part, at least–for blocking disease-causing pathogens from entering the blood stream. The circulatory system distributes vital substances through the body. The lymphatic system sends leaked fluids from the cardiovascular system back to the blood vessels. The reproductive system stores bodily hormones that influence gender traits.

18. D: The *parasympathetic nerves* are active when an individual is either resting or eating. The sympathetic nerves are active when an individual experiences a strong emotion, such as fear or excitement. Feeling pain and heat fall under the responsibility of the sensory neurons. Talking and walking fall under the responsibility of the ganglia within the sensory-somatic nervous system.

19. A: The integumentary system (i.e., the skin, hair, mucous, etc.) coordinates with the circulatory system to remove excess heat from the body. The superficial blood vessels (those nearest the surface of the skin) dilate to allow the heat to exit the body. The hormonal influence on blood pressure is the result of the relationship between the circulatory system and the endocrine system. The urinary system is responsible for assisting in the regulation of blood's pressure and volume. The skeletal system is responsible for assisting in the development of blood vessels within the marrow.

20. B: After the blood has gone through the left atrium, it enters the mitral valve before entering the left ventricle.

21. D: There are three domains: Archaea, Eukarya, and Eubacteria. *Fungi*, along with Plantae, Animalia, and Protista, falls within the Eukarya domain.

22. A: Cytokines signal to cells that damaged tissues need to be repaired. Perforins specifically target viruses and cancers. Leukocytes are the white blood cells that respond when tissues need to be repaired. Interferons help in the response to virus attacks by keeping the virus from replicating and spreading within the body.

23. B: The vacuoles function as a type of storage unit cell needs. In plant cells, the vacuoles are larger than in eukaryotic cells due to the water content that they require for adequate cell pressure.

24. C: The S phase is the third phase of interphase during mitosis.

25. C: The code is composed of the substances within DNA: adenine (A), cytosine (C), guanine (G), and thymine (T). It is possible to make 64 codons from the combination of these letters.

26. A: Ultraviolet light can cause the genetic mutations. Phosphate is a natural part of DNA, as are proteins. In fact, it is the alteration of the natural phosphate structure of the DNA that results in a mutation. Nucleotides also form a natural base within DNA.

27. C: The equation for photosynthesis requires a combination of carbon dioxide (CO_2), water, and sunlight to result in glucose and oxygen.

28. D: The vaccine brings a small amount of an infection into the body to give the body a chance to build up defenses to it by producing antibodies. These antibodies will recognize the disease in the future and prevent contraction of it.

29. B: The substance thymine cannot exist in RNA.

30. C: The substance *uracil* exists in RNA, in place of thymine.

31. A: Scientists have found that fertility rates tend to decrease as societies become more industrialized. As a result, the most industrialized countries typically have low fertility rates, while the least industrialized countries have higher fertility rates. With this in mind, and considering the information provided, Namibia--the least industrialized in the list of nations that is provided--can be expected to have the highest fertility rates.

32. D: Question 32 presents the theory of *natural selection*, or Darwin's theory of the *survival of the fittest*: individuals within a species develop characteristics that allow them to survive and reproduce more effectively (passing on the genes that they carry).

33. B: Each gene must match to a protein for a genetic trait to develop correctly.

34. D: The only true statement among the answer choices is that the majority of mutations are spontaneous. Very few mutations result from disease (although some diseases might result from genetic mutation). Some mutations (such as hemophilia) are indeed hereditary, so they can be passed on through the generations. Harmful chemicals are a known source of genetic mutations, so mutations that result from this source cannot be considered rare.

35. C: Protons are positively charged and found within the nucleus of an atom, while electrons are negatively charged and are found around the nucleus.

36. D: Solids with a fixed shape have a crystalline order that defines and maintains that shape.

37. D: A hydrogen atom creates a weak bond in DNA--in fact, this weak bond is known as a hydrogen bond due to the presence of the hydrogen atom.

38. B: The endoplasmic reticulum is the cell's transport network that moves proteins from one part of the cell to another. The Golgi apparatus assists in the transport but is not the actual transport network. Mitochondria are organelles ("tiny organs") that help in the production of ATP, which the cells need to operate properly. The nucleolus participates in the production of ribosomes that are needed to generate proteins for the cell.

39. A: The chromosomes separate during anaphase and move to the opposite ends of the cells.

40. C: Gamma rays are the shortest wavelengths in the spectrum. From longest to shortest: radio, microwave, infrared, visible, ultraviolet, x-ray, gamma.

41. D: Adenine is the fourth type of nitrogenous base in DNA. Bromine is not part of DNA construction. Uracil is found in RNA but not in DNA.

42. C: The Law of Conservation of Energy states that energy is never actually lost but instead is transferred back and forth from kinetic to potential. Answer choices A and B do not make much sense, and answer choice D reflects Newton's Second Law instead of the Law of Conservation of Energy.

43. A: The physical expression--such as hair color--is the result of the phenotype. The genotype is the basic genetic code.

44. B: Charge and isotope do not affect the number of protons: protons are determined by the atomic number as shown in the periodic table. Nitrogen (N) has an atomic number of 7, so that is the number of protons that a negatively charted isotope of N-12 has.

45. C: An ion results from an imbalance of charges on an atom after a reaction. A neutral atom has an equal number of protons and electrons so the number of positive charges from the protons is balanced by the amount of negative charges from the electrons. When electrons are transferred between atoms during a chemical reaction, an atom will become positively charged if it has lost electrons or negatively charged if it has gained electrons.

46. C: The number of 7 is the "breaking point" between basic and acidic. Above 7 solutions are considered basic; below 7 solutions are considered acidic. For instance, milk, with a pH of 6.5, is actually considered acidic. Bleach, with a pH of 12.5, is considered basic.

47. B: Mutations result from mutagen-induced changes or errors during DNA replication. That being said, DNA replication is a normal activity, so answer choice A cannot be said to cause mutations. Similarly, excision repair (answer choice C) and the presence of germ cells (answer choice D) are normal within DNA, so neither causes mutations. Errors that occur during these processes, however, might.

48. A: Scientists measure the distance between the earth and the stars (including the sun) in light-years, which is calculated as the distance that light will travel in one year.

49. D: Potential energy is energy that *can* be used but is not currently being used. A ballerina doing stretches is using energy. A secretary typing at a computer is also using energy. Note that a great deal of energy does not have to be used for the energy to be considered *kinetic* or in use (as a result of motion). A ball being thrown from one person to another is in motion and thus possesses kinetic energy. A rubber band stretched to its fullest and held, however, is waiting to spring back and possesses *potential* energy, or the energy that is being stored before use.

50. C: RNA has several roles, one of which is to act as the messenger and deliver information about the correct sequence of proteins in DNA. The ribosomes do the actual manufacturing of the proteins. Hydrogen, oxygen, and nitrogen work to create the bonds within DNA. And far from having a double helix shape, RNA has what would be considered a more two-dimensional shape.

51. B: Catalysts alter the activation energy during a chemical reaction and therefore control the rate of the reaction. The substrate is the actual surface that enzymes use during a chemical reaction (and there is no such term as *substrate energy*). Inhibitors and promoters participate in the chemical reaction, but it is the activation energy that catalysts alter to control the overall rate as the reaction occurs.

52. D: A metallic ion is called a *cation*, while a nonmetallic ion is called an *anion*. *Metalloid* refers to a type of element that easily accepts or gives off electrons. The term *covalent* refers to a specific type of bond between elements (that is, when atoms share electrons).

53. D: An *alkene* has a double bond, while an *alkyne* has a triple bond. The *alkane* is the saturated hydrocarbon that is altered to produce the unsaturated hydrocarbons with the double or triple bonds. For instance, ethane is the alkane; ethene is the alkene; ethyne is the alkyne.

54. C: Crossing the corresponding alleles from each parent will yield a result of BB in the upper right box of this Punnett square.

English and Language Usage Answer Explanations

1. C: The word *syllabi* is the correct plural form of *syllabus*. The other answer choices reflect incorrect plural forms. Specifically, *syllabus* does not change the form at all, and the Latin root of *syllabus* would require some change. At the same time, *syllaba*--while an accurate plural for some words with Latin roots--is incorrect in this case. And *syllabis* is a double form of the plural, so it cannot be correct.

2. A: The word *independent* is an adjective that modifies the word *state*, describing the type of state that described the kingdom of Gwynedd. The words *century*, *government*, and *control* are all nouns in this context.

3. B: Correct subject-verb agreement would require the singular verb *is* to accompany the singular subject *Big Island*. Readers should not be distracted by the use of *islands* in the appositive phrase just before the verb. The subject-verb relationship is governed by the word that functions as the subject of the sentence, instead of the noun (or, in some cases, the pronoun) that is closest to the verb.

4. C: Answer choice A is correct, because the quotation is a standard quotation (requiring double quotes) as well as a question. Additionally, the question mark belongs inside the quotation marks. Answer choice A correctly places the question mark inside the quotation marks, but the use of single quotes is incorrect for standard quotations. Answer choice B is incorrect, because it places the question mark outside the quotation marks. Answer choice D uses the layered quotes, which are unnecessary in this case, since the sentence presents only one quotation instead of more than one.

5. A: The word *its* is a possessive pronoun the reflects the collar belonging to the dog, and the use of *his* applies to Cody. Answer choice B incorrectly uses the contraction for *it is*. Answer choice C switches the pronouns so that *its* refers to Cody instead of the dog. Answer choice D does the same thing, except with the contraction for *it is* instead of the possessive pronoun.

6. D: *acceptable* is the correct spelling of the word. All other forms represent incorrect spelling of a commonly misspelled word.

7. C: Answer choice C offers the most effective combination of the sentences with the use of the conjunction *but* and the dependent clause starting with *after*. All other answer choices result in choppy or unclear combinations of the four sentences.

8. A: The original sentence contains two passive usages (*was expected* and *would be canceled*). Neither is necessary; both can be adjusted to improve the clarity of the sentence. Answer choice A best adjusts the passive tense to active. Answer choice B awkwardly makes *snow* the subject of the sentence when *administration* is a more effective subject. Answer choice C simply replaces *by* with *among*, but this does nothing to improve the clarity of the sentence. Answer choice D offers a nominalization (*expectation*), which clutters the sentence instead of improves it.

9. A: Correct punctuation requires a comma after both city and state when both fall within the sentence, even when the city and state fall within an opening dependent clause that has a comma after it. All answer choices that do not have a comma after the state as well as the city are incorrect. Answer choice C is incorrect because it adds a comma after *Oak* for no clear reason as the name of the city in full is clearly *Oak Ridge*.

10. C: The word *council* is a collective noun that, in this case, represents a group of individuals functioning individually. As a result, *council* is plural, so it needs the plural pronoun *they*. Within the context of the sentence, *he and she* makes no sense, and *each* is singular in this case, so it does not indicate the plural nature of the council.

11. A: The suffix *-ism* here suggests a doctrine that is followed, whether that be the doctrine of polytheism (a religious doctrine), communism (a social doctrine), or nationalism (a political doctrine).

12. B: Question 12 asks for the correct punctuation of layered quotations. Standard American usage requires the double quotes for the first quotation and the single quotes for any quotes within the original quotes. Answer choice B best reflects this with the phrase "Let there be light" representing the quote within the original quotation. Answer choice A reverses the correct usage. Answer choice C incorrectly makes the entire quotation a quote within an otherwise unidentified quote. Answer choice D uses double quotes within the double quotes, which is incorrect in standard American usage.

13. D: The semicolon correctly joins the two sentences. Answer choice A is incorrect, because it uses a comma splice to join two independent clauses. (To join two independent clauses, a comma needs to be accompanied by a coordinating conjunction.) The colon in answer choice B is incorrect because the information in the second clause does not clearly define or explain the previous clause. Answer choice C is incorrect because it offers no punctuation to separate the two independent clauses and thus creates more confusion than clarity.

14. C: Question 14 asks the student to identify and remove the nominalization. In the original sentence, the nominalization is *commitment*. The easiest way to remove the nominalization is to adjust it to the verb *commit*. As a result, answer choice C is the only correct option because it identifies and removes the nominalization.

15. B: Answer choice B contains two independent clauses that are joined with a comma and the coordinating conjunction *and*. Answer choice A, though it contains a compound subject and a compound verb, is still a simple sentence. Answer choice C opens within a dependent clause, so it is a complex sentence. Answer choice D is a compound-complex sentence because it includes a dependent clause as well as two independent clauses.

16. B: Answer choice B correctly capitalizes *Uncle Archibald*, where *Uncle* refers to a specific name. The word *cousin* needs no capitalization, even when it refers to the name of a specific relative. (The only distinctions are when the word is used within a direct address or opens a sentence.) Similarly, *mother* and *sister* do not need to be capitalized unless they are the first word of the sentence or are part of a direct address.

17. B: The word *count* is part of an infinitive phrase (*to count*), and infinitive phrases function as nouns, so the word *count* cannot be a verb. All other answer choices are verbs.

18. D: The word *affect* is a verb in this context and is the correct usage within the sentence. The possessive pronoun *your* also correctly modifies *children*, so answer choice D is correct. All other answer choices incorrectly apply the words to the sentence.

19. B: The context of the sentence suggests that the trauma of surviving the plane crash left long-term memories that haunted Johanna for many years. As a result, *permanent* is the best meaning of *indelible*. The other meanings make little sense in the context of the sentence. The only possible option is *indirect*, but there is nothing about the sentence to suggest that the nightmares are indirect impressions of a traumatic experience.

20. C: The word *east* in answer choice C is simply a directional indication and does not need to be capitalized in the context of the sentence. All other uses of capitalization are correct in the context of the sentences. The word *South* should be capitalized when it refers to a region of the United States (as indicated by the mention of Mississippi). The word *East* should be capitalized when it refers to the region of Texas. And the word *north* does not need to be capitalized when it is simply a directional indication (as in answer choice D).

21. A: The word *phenomena* is the correct plural form of *phenomenon*, so answer choice A is correct. The correct plural form of *mother-in-law* is *mothers-in-law*. The correct plural form of *deer* is just *deer*. The correct plural form of *roof* is *roofs*.

22. C: The word *whom* correctly indicates the objective case--as in "to hold him/her responsible"--so answer choice C is correct. The word *who* in answer choice A incorrectly indicates the subjective case. Similarly, answer choice B is incorrect because the word *who* is the subjective case (instead of the objective case) here. Answer choice D is incorrect because it incorrect applies the objective *whom* instead of the subjective *who*.

23. B: The word *capacity* is a noun in this context, so answer choice B is correct. Because the word functions as the object of the preposition, the options of verb and adverb cannot be correct. Answer choice D is incorrect because the word *capacity* is not a pronoun in any context.

24. C: Answer choice C summarizes the ideas within the sentence simply and clearly. Answer choice A moves the ideas around to make them awkward instead of effective. Answer choice B creates a dangling modifier with the phrase *without adequate protection*, so it cannot be correct. Similarly, answer choice D makes this phrase a dangling modifier that makes the flow of thought awkward instead of clear.

25. D: The context of the sentence suggests that the word *exorbitant* refers to an excessively high cost, so answer choice D is most correct. Answer choice A would be an interesting conclusion to the sentence, but it does not clearly follow the use of *exorbitant*, so it cannot be correct. Answer choices B and C contradict the suggested meaning of *exorbitant*, so both must be incorrect.

26. A: The pronoun *all* is plural, so it requires the plural verb *are*. The pronouns *each* and *neither* are singular and require singular verbs (not provided in answer choices B and C). The pronoun *any* can be either singular or plural depending on the context of the sentence. In this case, *any* suggests a singular usage, so answer choice D is incorrect with the plural verb.

27. C: The pronouns *she and I* are correctly in the subjective case starting the second independent clause, so answer choice C is correct. All other answer choices contain at least one incorrect objective case usage that cannot function as the subject of the second independent clause.
28. A: Both *her* and *me* are objective case pronouns that accurately function as the object of the preposition *to*. All other answer choices contain at least one incorrect subjective case usage that cannot function as the object of the preposition.

29. D: While answer choice D is arguably the longest of the four sentences, it is actually a simple sentence. It contains a compound subject and a compound verb, but because it represents only one independent clause it still functions as a simple sentence. Answer choices A and B contain two independent clauses and are thus compound sentences. Answer choice C contains a dependent clause, so it is a complex sentence.

30. B: The word *President* should always be capitalized when it refers to the President of the United States, whether or not the President's name is included. All other nouns in this sentence are simple nouns and do not need to be capitalized.

31. C: The word *playwright* is the correct spelling to refer to someone who writes plays. All other forms are incorrect and reflect common confusion about the correct spelling of the word.

32. D: Answer choice D correctly arranges the ideas to reflect the most effective meaning of the sentence. All other answer choices place the ideas in such a way as to create confusion or incorrect punctuation instead of clarity and correctness.

33. C: In the context, the collective noun *jury* reflects a unit functioning as one, so the word is singular instead of plural. Answer choice C, the singular possessive pronoun *its*, is correct, while answer choice D (the plural *their*) cannot be correct. The word *it's* is the contraction for *it is*. The word *they're* is the contraction for *they are*.

34. A: Answer choice A correctly places the word *compliment* to refer to Amber's positive remark and *complement* to refer to the excellent way that the pieces of furniture work together.

TEAS® Practice Test #2

Reading	Mathematics	Science		English and Language Usage
1. _____	1. _____	1. _____	49. _____	1. _____
2. _____	2. _____	2. _____	50. _____	2. _____
3. _____	3. _____	3. _____	51. _____	3. _____
4. _____	4. _____	4. _____	52. _____	4. _____
5. _____	5. _____	5. _____	53. _____	5. _____
6. _____	6. _____	6. _____	54. _____	6. _____
7. _____	7. _____	7. _____		7. _____
8. _____	8. _____	8. _____		8. _____
9. _____	9. _____	9. _____		9. _____
10. _____	10. _____	10. _____		10. _____
11. _____	11. _____	11. _____		11. _____
12. _____	12. _____	12. _____		12. _____
13. _____	13. _____	13. _____		13. _____
14. _____	14. _____	14. _____		14. _____
15. _____	15. _____	15. _____		15. _____
16. _____	16. _____	16. _____		16. _____
17. _____	17. _____	17. _____		17. _____
18. _____	18. _____	18. _____		18. _____
19. _____	19. _____	19. _____		19. _____
20. _____	20. _____	20. _____		20. _____
21. _____	21. _____	21. _____		21. _____
22. _____	22. _____	22. _____		22. _____
23. _____	23. _____	23. _____		23. _____
24. _____	24. _____	24. _____		24. _____
25. _____	25. _____	25. _____		25. _____
26. _____	26. _____	26. _____		26. _____
27. _____	27. _____	27. _____		27. _____
28. _____	28. _____	28. _____		28. _____
29. _____	29. _____	29. _____		29. _____
30. _____	30. _____	30. _____		30. _____
31. _____	31. _____	31. _____		31. _____
32. _____	32. _____	32. _____		32. _____
33. _____	33. _____	33. _____		33. _____
34. _____	34. _____	34. _____		34. _____
35. _____		35. _____		
36. _____		36. _____		
37. _____		37. _____		
38. _____		38. _____		
39. _____		39. _____		
40. _____		40. _____		
41. _____		41. _____		
42. _____		42. _____		
43. _____		43. _____		
44. _____		44. _____		
45. _____		45. _____		
46. _____		46. _____		
47. _____		47. _____		
48. _____		48. _____		

Section 1. Reading

1. At first, the woman's contractions were only intermittent, so the nurse had trouble determining how far her labor had progressed. Which of the following is the definition for the underlined word?
    a. frequent
    b. irregular
    c. painful
    d. dependable

2. Fearful that the patron might burn himself, Edith made sure to say, "**Hot plate**, sir" when she set the dish on his table. The use of bold font in the text above indicates which of the following?
    a. dialogue
    b. emphasis
    c. thoughts
    d. anger

3. Students who pursue a degree in a humanities discipline (e.g., English, history, philosophy, art, film studies) often have a difficult time finding work after they graduate. Which of the following does the abbreviation "e.g." stand for?
    a. error
    b. correction
    c. addition
    d. example

4. The guide words at the top of a dictionary page are *needs* and *negotiate*. Which of the following words is an entry on this page?
    a. needle
    b. neigh
    c. neglect
    d. nectar

5. Chapter 4: The Fictional Writings of Dorothy L. Sayers
    Plays
    Novels
    Short Stories
    Letters
    Mysteries

Analyze the headings above. Which of the following does not belong?
    a. Novels
    b. Plays
    c. Mysteries
    d. Letters

Among the first females awarded a degree from Oxford University, Dorothy L. Sayers proved to be one of the most versatile writers in post-war England. Sayers was born in 1893, the only child of an Anglican chaplain, and she received an unexpectedly good education at home. For instance, her study of Latin commenced when she was only six years old. She entered Oxford in 1912, at a time when the university was not granting degrees to women. By 1920, this policy had changed, and Sayers received her degree in medieval literature and modern languages after finishing university. That same year, she also received a master of arts degree.

Sayers's first foray into published writing was a collection of poetry released in 1916. Within a few years, she began work on the detective novels and short stories that would make her famous, due to the creation of the foppish, mystery-solving aristocrat Lord Peter Wimsey. Sayers is also credited with the short story mysteries about the character Montague Egg. In spite of her success as a mystery writer, Sayers continued to balance popular fiction with academic work; her translation of Dante's *Inferno* gained her respect for her ability to convey the poetry in English while still remaining true to the Italian *terza rima*. She also composed a series of twelve plays about the life of Christ, and wrote several essays about education and feminism. In her middle age, Dorothy L. Sayers published several works of Christian apologetics, one of which was so well-received that the archbishop of Canterbury attempted to present her with a doctorate of divinity. Sayers, for reasons known only to her, declined.

The next three questions are based on the above passage.

6. Which of the following describes the type of writing used to create the passage?
   a. narrative
   b. persuasive
   c. expository
   d. technical

7. Which of the following sentences is the best summary of the passage?
   a. Among the first females awarded a degree from Oxford University, Dorothy L. Sayers proved to be one of the most versatile writers in post-war England.
   b. Sayers was born in 1893, the only child of an Anglican chaplain, and she received an unexpectedly good education at home.
   c. Within a few years, she began work on the detective novels and short stories that would make her famous, due to the creation of the foppish, mystery-solving aristocrat Lord Peter Wimsey.
   d. In her middle age, Dorothy L. Sayers published several works of Christian apologetics, one of which was so well-received that the archbishop of Canterbury attempted to present her with a doctorate of divinity.

8. Which of the following sentences contains an opinion statement by the author?
   a. Among the first females awarded a degree from Oxford University, Dorothy L. Sayers proved to be one of the most versatile writers in post-war England.
   b. Sayers was born in 1893, the only child of an Anglican chaplain, and she received an unexpectedly good education at home.
   c. Her translation of Dante's Inferno gained her respect for her ability to convey the poetry in English while still remaining true to the Italian terza rima.
   d. Sayers, for reasons known only to her, declined.

The Dewey Decimal Classes
000 Computer science, information, and general works
100 Philosophy and psychology
200 Religion
300 Social sciences
400 Languages
500 Science and mathematics
600 Technical and applied science
700 Arts and recreation
800 Literature
900 History, geography, and biography

The next four questions are based on the above information.

9. Jorgen is doing a project on the ancient Greek mathematician and poet Eratosthenes. In his initial review, Jorgen learns that Eratosthenes is considered the first person to calculate the circumference of the earth, and that he is considered the first to describe geography as it is studied today. To which section of the library should Jorgen go to find one of the early maps created by Eratosthenes?
   a. 100
   b. 300
   c. 600
   d. 900

10. Due to his many interests and pursuits, Eratosthenes dabbled in a variety of fields, and he is credited with a theory known as the sieve of Eratosthenes. This is an early algorithm used to determine prime numbers. To which section of the library should Jorgen go to find out more about the current applications of the sieve of Eratosthenes?
   a. 000
   b. 100
   c. 400
   d. 500

11. One ancient work claims that Eratosthenes received the nickname "beta" from those who knew him. This is a word that represents the second letter of the Greek alphabet, and it represented Eratosthenes's accomplishments in every area that he studied. To which section of the library should Jorgen go to learn more about the letters of the Greek alphabet and the meaning of the word "beta"?
   a. 200
   b. 400
   c. 700
   d. 900

12. Finally, Jorgen learns that Eratosthenes was fascinated by the story of the Trojan War, and that he attempted to determine the exact dates when this event occurred. Jorgen is unfamiliar with the story of the Fall of Troy, so he decides to look into writings such as *The Iliad* and *The Odyssey*, by Homer. To which section of the library should Jorgen go to locate these works?
   a. 100
   b. 200
   c. 700
   d. 800

13. With all of the planning that preceded her daughter's wedding, Marci decided that picking out a new paint color for her own living room was largely <u>peripheral</u>. Which of the following is the definition for the underlined word?
    a. meaningless
    b. contrived
    c. unimportant
    d. disappointing

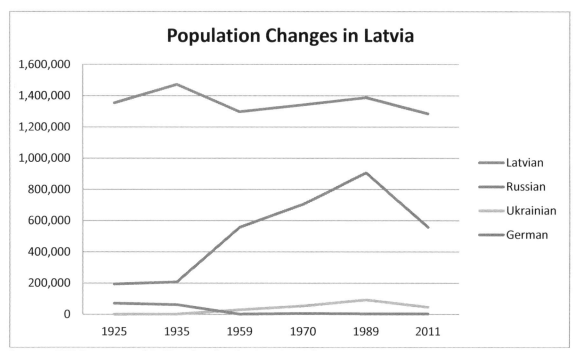

Source: UN Demographic Yearbooks / minorityrights.org

The next four questions are based on the chart above, which reflects the population changes in Latvia during the 20th century as shown through four ethnic groups (Latvian, Russian, Ukrainian, and German).

14. In 2011, the population of Latvia was just over two million people. Of the four ethnic groups shown on the chart above, which represented approximately 25 percent of the total population of Latvia in 2011?
    a. Latvian
    b. Russian
    c. Ukrainian
    d. German

15. According to the chart above, which of the following ethnic groups had the largest percent decrease in population between 1925 and 2011?
    a. Latvian
    b. Russian
    c. Ukrainian
    d. German

16. Between 1925 and 1991, Latvia was part of the Soviet Union. Since 1991, the population of which ethnic group in Latvia appears to have decreased the most?
   a. Latvian
   b. Russian
   c. Ukrainian
   d. German

17. After World War II ended in 1945, large numbers of non-Latvian workers entered the country, primarily to work at construction jobs. Among these non-Latvian ethnic groups, the increase in workers represented a population percentage shift of less than one percent before 1945 to more than three percent by the time of the Soviet Union's collapse. Which ethnic group shown on the chart best represents this shift?
   a. Latvian
   b. Russian
   c. Ukrainian
   d. German

18. Follow the numbered instructions to transform the starting word into a different word.
   1. Start with the word CORPOREAL.
   2. Remove the C from the beginning of the word.
   3. Remove the O from the beginning of the word.
   4. Remove the O from the middle of the word.
   5. Move the E to follow the first R.
   6. Move the L to follow the P.
   7. Remove the second R.
   8. Add the letter Y to the end of the word.

What is the new word?
   a. REALLY
   b. PRETTY
   c. REPLAY
   d. POWER

19. Although not considered the smartest student in her class, Klara was willing to work hard for her grades, and her <u>sedulous</u> commitment to her studies earned her top scores at graduation. Which of the following is the definition for the underlined word?
   a. diligent
   b. silent
   c. moderate
   d. complicated

20. Flemming is on a new diet that requires him to avoid all dairy products, as well as dairy byproducts. This will be a big change for him, so his doctor gives him information about foods that he might not realize often contain dairy products. These include the following: bread and bread crumbs, granola, deli meat, dry breakfast cereal, and energy bars. Which of the following items from Flemming's standard diet will still be safe to eat?
   a. puffed rice cereal
   b. breaded chicken parmesan
   c. sliced turkey sandwich
   d. yogurt made from coconut milk

Car Owner's Manual: Table of Contents:
   Vehicle Instruments
   Safety Options
   Audio, Climate, and Voice Controls
   Pre-Driving and Driving
   Routine Maintenance
   Emergencies
   Consumer Resources

The next four questions are based on the above information.

21. To which chapter should Regina turn if she needs to locate information about adjusting the air conditioning in the vehicle?
   a. I
   b. II
   c. III
   d. IV

22. To which chapter should Regina turn if she needs to find out how often the car manufacturer recommends having the oil changed?
   a. IV
   b. V
   c. VI
   d. VII

23. To which chapter should Regina turn if she wants to find out where the nearest dealership is located?
   a. I
   b. III
   c. V
   d. VII

24. To which chapter should Regina turn if she needs to find out what to do if the car begins overheating?
   a. II
   b. III
   c. IV
   d. VI

25. Nora is preparing a large research project for the end of the term, and the instructor has required that all students make sure they are using reliable, scholarly resources in their papers. Of the following resource options, which would not be considered a reliable, scholarly source?
    a. Encyclopedia Britannica
    b. Wikipedia
    c. Science.gov
    d. LexisNexis

26. In Sonnet 18, Shakespeare wrote, "Shall I compare thee to a summer's day? / Thou art more lovely and more temperate."
Which of the following is the definition for the underlined word in the sentence above?
    a. modest
    b. conservative
    c. agreeable
    d. immoderate

27. In the sonnet quoted above, what does the slash between the sentences represent?
    a. the end of one stanza and the beginning of another
    b. the end of a question and the answer that follows
    c. the end of one line of poetry and the start of the next
    d. the end of one sentence and the start of the next

The Big Book of Herbs and Herbal Medicine

The next four questions are based on the above information.

28. Clothilde is looking for an herbal remedy to combat a recent outbreak of eczema. In which chapter should she look for more information?
    a. Chapter 8
    b. Chapter 10
    c. Chapter 11
    d. Chapter 12

29. Clothilde's sister has asked her to recommend an herbal therapy for her five-year-old daughter's chronic cough. In which chapter should Clothilde look for more information?
    a. Chapter 7
    b. Chapter 9
    c. Chapter 10
    d. Chapter 12

30. Clothilde's elderberry plant is nearly overgrown, and she is hoping to trim it back and use the elderflower to prepare a blend of tea, as well as a homemade wine. In which chapter should she look for more information about how to do this?
   a. Chapter 3
   b. Chapter 4
   c. Chapter 5
   d. Chapter 13

31. Clothilde realizes that she failed to maintain her elderberry plant as she should have, and she needs tips about how to keep the plant in good condition to avoid another overgrowth. In which chapter should she look for more information?
   a. Chapter 2
   b. Chapter 3
   c. Chapter 13
   d. Chapter 14

> **LOOKING FOR ROOMMATE – CLEAN HOUSE / QUIET AREA / CLOSE TO UNIVERSITY**
> Need one more female roommate for 3-bd house w/in walking distance of univ. Current occupants quiet, house clean/smoke-free. No pets. Long-term applicants preferred. Rent: $800/mo. Utilities/Internet included. Avail: Aug 15. Call Florence at 985-5687, or send an email to f.carpenter@email.com.

32. Florence receives a number of calls about the roommate advertisement. Of the individuals described below, who seems like the best applicant?
   a. Frances is a research assistant in the science department who has a Yorkshire terrier.
   b. Adelaide works in the humanities department and is looking for a three-month rental.
   c. Cosette is allergic to cigarette smoke and needs a quiet place to study.
   d. Felix is a graduate student in the history department who doesn't have a car.

---

33. Performing Arts in Museville
     Music
     Opera
     Sculpture
     Dance
     Theater
     Film

Analyze the headings above. Which of the following does not belong?
   a. Opera
   b. Sculpture
   c. Film
   d. Music

COMPANY	ENGLISH BREAKFAST	EARL GREY	DARJEELING	OOLONG	GREEN
Tea Heaven	$25	$27	$26	$32	$30
Wholesale Tea	$24	$24	$24	$26	$27
Tea by The Pound	$22	$25	$30	$28	$29
Tea Express	$25	$28	$26	$29	$30

Note: Prices per 16 oz. (1 pound)

The next two questions are based on the above table.

34. Noella runs a small tea shop and needs to restock. She is running very low on English Breakfast and Darjeeling tea, and she needs two pounds of each. Which company can offer her the best price on the two blends?
   a. Tea Heaven
   b. Wholesale Tea
   c. Tea by The Pound
   d. Tea Express

35. After reviewing her inventory, Noella realizes that she also needs one pound of Earl Grey and two pounds of green tea. Which company can offer her the best price on these two blends?
   a. Tea Heaven
   b. Wholesale Tea
   c. Tea by The Pound
   d. Tea Express

36. The United Nations Statistics Division has divided the continent of Europe into four primary areas: Northern Europe, Southern Europe, Western Europe, and Eastern Europe. Northern Europe is comprised of eleven nations that make up Scandinavia, the Baltic states, and Great Britain. According to this definition, which of the following capital cities would not be located in Northern Europe?
   a. Copenhagen
   b. Oslo
   c. London
   d. Kiev

37. The United Nations Statistics Division loosely defines Southern Europe as the area made up of the nations that border the Mediterranean Sea (with the exception of France, which is considered part of Western Europe) and the Black Sea. The single exception to this definition is a nation on the Iberian Peninsula, which borders the Atlantic Ocean but has no Mediterranean coastline. The Iberian Peninsula is also home to Spain, Andorra, and Gibraltar. Which of the following is the other, non-Mediterranean nation on the Iberian Peninsula?
   a. Portugal
   b. Bulgaria
   c. Italy
   d. Cyprus

Dear library patrons:

To ensure that all visitors have the opportunity to use our limited number of computers, we ask that each person restrict himself or herself to 30 minutes on a computer. For those needing to use a computer beyond this time frame, there will be a $3 charge for each 15-minute period.

We thank you in advance for your cooperation.

Pineville Library

The next two questions are based on the above information.

38. Which of the following is a logical conclusion that can be derived from the announcement above?
    a. The library is planning to purchase more computers, but cannot afford them yet.
    b. The library is facing budget cuts, and is using the Internet fee to compensate for them.
    c. The library has added the fee to discourage patrons from spending too long on the computers.
    d. The library is offsetting its own Internet service costs by passing on the fee to patrons.

39. Raoul has an upcoming school project, and his own computer is not working. He needs to use the library computer, and he has estimated that he will need to be on the computer for approximately an hour and a half. How much of a fee can Raoul expect to pay for his computer use at the library?
    a. $6
    b. $9
    c. $12
    d. $15

371 SALON AND SPA SERVICES

Hair Salons

Angel Cuts 118 Sparrow	(345) 485-5717
Hair and a Spare 274 Finch	
Extensions	
Handmade Wigs	(345) 485-5547
Perfect Endings 687 Canary	(345) 485-5524
Quick Trims 824 Parakeet	(345) 485-7569

Nail Salons

Hands to Envy 148 Canary	(345) 485-2138
Nails by Manhattan 958 Avocet	(345) 485-6748
Natural Nails 285 Finch	(345) 485-7691

Tanning Salons

Airbrushed Tans 687 Avocet	(345) 485-9482
Cannes Tan 812 Kittiwake	(587) 785-5875
Paparazzi-Ready Tans 885 Sparrow	(345) 485-4812
Spray Tans Unlimited 671 Grouse	(345) 485-7595

Salon and Spa Services

Good Karma Salon & Spa 448 Ptarmigan	
Haircuts, Styling, Coloring	
Nails, Tanning, Massages	(345) 485-7824
Holistic Health 986 Teal	
Natural Health & Wellness	(345) 485-3333
Sérénité Spa 875 Tanager	
Full-Body Relaxation	(345) 485-5846
Total Wellness Day Spa 264 Avocet	
Full Spa Svcs Available	(345) 485-8795

CANNES TAN
...WHEN YOU CAN'T MAKE IT TO THE RIVIERA
587-785-5875

Angel Cuts
"The Best Haircut in Town"
345-485-5717
Check our website for coupons!

Sérénité Spa – NOW OPEN!
Offering full-body relaxation in a state-of-the-art spa. All spa services available. Call for an appointment with one of our trained aestheticians today!
345-485-5845

Natural Nails
All-Natural Nail Services
-- No harsh chemicals
-- No toxic products
345-485-7691

Hair and a Spare
The best local salon for extensions and wigs made just for you! Satisfaction guaranteed. Call today to set up an appointment. Be sure to ask for our first-time customer discount!
(345) 485-5547

The next three questions are based on the above information.

40. Genevieve has recently moved to the area, and she is looking for a salon where she can get a haircut and color, as well as a manicure and pedicure for an upcoming event. Based on the information above, which location is most likely to offer all of these services?
    a. Sérénité Spa
    b. Angel Cuts
    c. Perfect Endings
    d. Good Karma Salon & Spa

41. After considering her options, Genevieve realizes she needs to be careful about where she gets her manicure and pedicure. The last time she had her nails done, she developed an allergic reaction to the nail polish that was used. With this in mind, which location might be the best choice?
    a. Nails by Manhattan
    b. Perfect Endings
    c. Natural Nails
    d. Hands to Envy

42. Based on the addresses shown on the phonebook page, which two businesses are likely in the same shopping center?
    a. Hair and a Spare and Natural Nails
    b. Perfect Endings and Hands to Envy
    c. Nails by Manhattan and Airbrushed Tans
    d. Angel Cuts and Cannes Tan

For lunch, she likes ham and cheese (torn into bites), yogurt, raisins, applesauce, peanut butter sandwiches in the fridge drawer, or any combo of these. She's not a huge eater. Help yourself too. Bread is on counter if you want to make a sandwich.

It's fine if you want to go somewhere, leave us a note of where you are. Make sure she's buckled and drive carefully! Certain fast food places are fun if they have playgrounds and are indoors. It's probably too hot for playground, but whatever you want to do is fine. Take a sippy cup of water and a diaper wherever you go. There's some money here for you in case you decide to go out for lunch with her.

As for nap, try after lunch. She may not sleep, but try anyway. Read her a couple of books first, put cream on her mosquito bites (it's in the den on the buffet), then maybe rock in her chair. Give her a bottle of milk, and refill as needed, but don't let her drink more than $2\frac{1}{2}$ bottles of milk or she'll throw up. Turn on music in her room, leave her in crib with a dry diaper and bottle to try to sleep. She likes a stuffed animal too. Try for 30-45 minutes. You may have to start the tape again. If she won't sleep, that's fine. We just call it "rest time" on those days that naps won't happen.

The next two questions are based on the above passage.

43. To whom is this passage probably being written?
    a. a mother
    b. a father
    c. a babysitter
    d. a nurse

44. You can assume the writer of the passage is:
    a. a mom
    b. a dad
    c. a teacher
    d. a parent

Volleyball is easy to learn and fun to play in a physical education class. With just one net and one ball, an entire class can participate. The object of the game is to get the ball over the net and onto the ground on the other side. At the same time, all players should be in the ready position to keep the ball from hitting the ground on their own side. After the ball has been served, the opposing team may have three hits to get the ball over the net to the other side. Only the serving team may score. If the receiving team wins the volley, the referee calls, "side out" and the receiving team wins the serve. Players should rotate positions so that everyone gets a chance to serve. A game is played to 15 points, but the winning team must win by two points. That means if the score is 14 to 15, the play continues until one team wins by two. A volleyball match consists of three games. The winner of the match is the team that wins two of the three games.

The next four questions are based on the above passage.

45. Who can score in a volleyball game?
    a. the receiving team
    b. the serving team
    c. either team
    d. there is no score

46. How many people can participate in a volleyball game?
    a. 14
    b. 15
    c. half of a class
    d. an entire class

47. What is something that a referee might call in a volleyball game?
    a. "side out"
    b. "time out"
    c. "out of order"
    d. "be careful"

48. What equipment is needed for volleyball?
    a. a referee, a goal, a ball
    b. a goal, a ball, a net
    c. a net, a ball
    d. two balls, one net

Section 2. Mathematics

1. Within a certain nursing program, 25% of the class wanted to work with infants, 60% of the class wanted to work with the elderly, 10% of the class wanted to assist general practitioners in private practices, and the rest were undecided. What fraction of the class wanted to work with the elderly?

    a. $\frac{1}{4}$

    b. $\frac{1}{10}$

    c. $\frac{3}{5}$

    d. $\frac{1}{20}$

2. Veronica has to create the holiday schedule for the neonatal unit at her hospital. She knows that 35% of the staff members will not be available because they are taking vacation days during the holiday. Of the remaining staff members who will be available, only 20% are certified to work in the neonatal unit. What percentage of the TOTAL staff is certified and available to work in the neonatal unit during the holiday?

    a. 7%

    b. 13%

    c. 65%

    d. 80%

3. A patient requires a 30% decrease in the dosage of his medication. His current dosage is 340 mg. What will his dosage be after the decrease?

    a. 70

    b. 238

    c. 270

    d. 340

4. A study about anorexia was conducted on 100 patients. Within that patient population 70% were women, and 10% of the men were overweight as children. How many male patients in the study were NOT overweight as children?

    a. 3

    b. 10

    c. 27

    d. 30

5. University Q has an extremely competitive nursing program. Historically, $\frac{3}{4}$ of the students in each incoming class major in nursing but only $\frac{1}{5}$ of those who major in nursing actually complete the program. If this year's incoming class has 100 students, how many students will complete the nursing program?

    a. 75

    b. 20

    c. 15

    d. 5

> Four nurse midwives take out small business loans to open a joint practice together. They use their loans to pay various expenses for the practice. Each nurse midwife receives $2000 per month.

The next five questions are based on the above information.

6. The first midwife uses $\frac{2}{5}$ of her loan to pay the rent and utilities for the office space. Then she divides the remainder in half so that she can save $\frac{1}{2}$ the remainder for incidental expenditures. She uses the rest of her loan to purchase medical supplies. How much money does she spend on medical supplies each month?

    a. $600

    b. $800

    c. $1000

    d. $1200

7. The second midwife budgets $\frac{1}{2}$ of her loan to pay an office administrator plus another $\frac{1}{10}$ of her loan for office supplies. What is the total fraction of the second midwife's small business loan that is spent on the office administrator and office supplies?

    a. $\frac{3}{5}$

    b. $\frac{2}{12}$

    c. $\frac{2}{20}$

    d. $\frac{1}{20}$

8. Each month, the third midwife pays $900 for malpractice insurance. Then she pays $200 for a cleaning service to sanitize the office. Finally, she pays $100 for advertising. How much money does the third midwife have left after paying these expenses?

    a. $1200

    b. $1100

    c. $900

    d. $800

9. The fourth midwife is saving to buy an office building for the practice. So each month she puts money aside in a special savings account. The ratio of her monthly savings to the rent is 1:2. If the rent is $800 per month, how much money does she put into the special savings account each month?
    a. $100
    b. $200
    c. $400
    d. $1600

10. All four midwives decided to combine their money to purchase an ultrasound machine. The first midwife gave $501.93 towards the purchase of the machine. The second contributed $498.05; the third gave $499.92, and the fourth gave $500.02. Estimate the total amount of money the midwives used to purchase the machine.
    a. $1000
    b. $1500
    c. $2000
    d. $2500

11. A patient was taking 310 mg of antidepressant each day. However, the doctor determined that this dosage was too high and reduced the dosage by 80 mg. What is the new dosage of the patient's antidepressant?
    a. 80 mg
    b. 230 mg
    c. 310 mg
    d. 390 mg

12. A lab technician took 100 hairs from a patient to conduct several tests. The technician used $\frac{1}{7}$ of the hairs for a drug test. How many hairs were used for the drug test? Round your answer to the nearest hundredth.
    a. 14.00
    b. 14.20
    c. 14.29
    d. 14.30

13. A patient was transferred from a hospital in Europe to an American hospital in order to receive a rare operation. The patient's medical chart lists his age in Roman numerals as XXIV. How old is the patient?
    a. 24
    b. 21
    c. 11
    d. 4

14. Susan is extremely excited about receiving her first job as a nurse. Her gross annual salary is $40,000. Susan contributes 10% of her salary **before** taxes to a retirement account. Then she pays 25% of her remaining salary in state and federal taxes. Finally, she pays $30 per month for health insurance. What is Susan's annual take-home pay?
   a. $25640
   b. $25970
   c. $26640
   d. $26970

15. Susan decided to celebrate getting her first nursing job by purchasing a new outfit. She bought a dress for $69.99 and a pair of shoes for $39.99. She also bought accessories for $34.67. What was the total cost of Susan's outfit, including accessories?
   a. $69.99
   b. $75.31
   c. $109.98
   d. $144.65

16. Use the following table from a checking account statement to determine the ending balance in the account.
   a. $88.50
   b. $239.16
   c. $300.00
   d. $511.50

Transaction description	Amount
Beginning balance	$300.00
Purchase coffee at cafe	$3.56
Pay utility bill	$132.61
Deposit money in ATM	$75.33
Ending balance	??

17. Complete the following equation:
$$2 + (2)(2) - 2 \div 2 = ?$$
   a. 5
   b. 3
   c. 2
   d. 1

18. The emergency room manager at a certain hospital will host a celebration for the doctors and staff because they met the quarterly wait-time goals. For each person who RSVPs for the celebration, the manager will order 2 cupcakes, 1 can of soda, and 1 serving of fruit salad. Each cupcake costs $1.75. A can of soda costs $0.75, and a serving of fruit salad costs $2.50. If 50 people RSVP for the event, how much will the emergency room manager spend on cupcakes?
   a. $87.50
   b. $125.00
   c. $175.00
   d. $337.50

19. As part of a study, a set of patients will be divided into three groups: $\frac{4}{15}$ of the patients will be in Group Alpha, $\frac{2}{5}$ of the patients will be in Group Beta, and $\frac{1}{3}$ of the patients will be in Group Gamma. Order the groups from smallest to largest, according to the number of patients in each group.
    a. Group Alpha, Group Beta, Group Gamma
    b. Group Alpha, Group Gamma, Group Beta
    c. Group Gamma, Group Alpha, Group Beta
    d. Group Gamma, Group Beta, Group Alpha

20. Solve the following equation:
$$2x + 6 = 14$$
    a. $x = 4$
    b. x = 8
    c. x = 10
    d. x = 13

21. Add polynomial #1 and polynomial #2.
                Polynomial #1: $4x + 2x + 2y + 4y$
                Polynomial #2: $8y + 6y + 4x + 2x$
    a. 12xy + 8xy + 6xy + 6xy
    b. 32xy
    c. 12y + 20x
    d. 12x + 20y

22. During week 1, Nurse Cameron worked 5 shifts. During week 2, she worked twice as many shifts as she did during week 1. During week 3, she added 4 shifts to the number of shifts she worked during week 2. Which equation below describes the number of shifts Nurse Cameron worked during week 3?
    a. shifts = (2)(5) + 4
    b. shifts = (4)(5) + 2
    c. shifts = 5 + 2 + 4
    d. shifts = (5)(2)(4)

23. Solve the following expression.
$$|(3)(-4)| + (3)(4) - 1$$
    a. -1
    b. 1
    c. 23
    d. 24

24. Which graph accurately describes the data presented in the table below?

Hospital Staff	Average hours worked per week
Administrators	40
Nurses	55
Residents	80
Physicians	35

a.

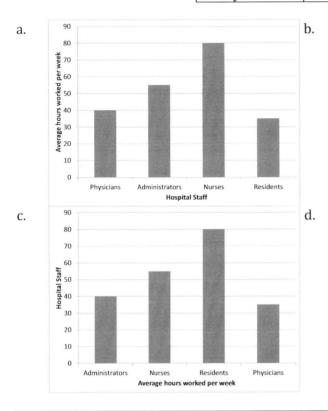

b.

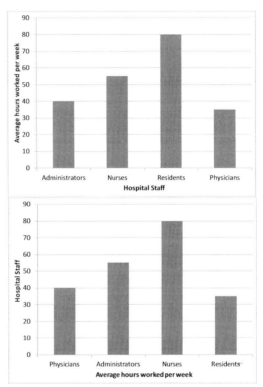

c.

d.

25. According to the circle graph below, which group works the most amount of time?

a. Residents
b. Physicians
c. Administrators
d. Nurses

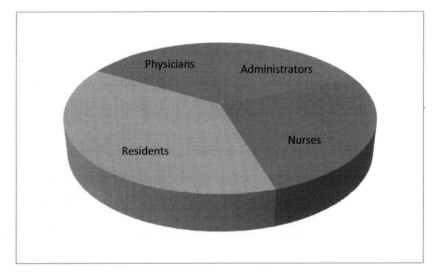

26. What are the dependent and independent variables in the graph below?

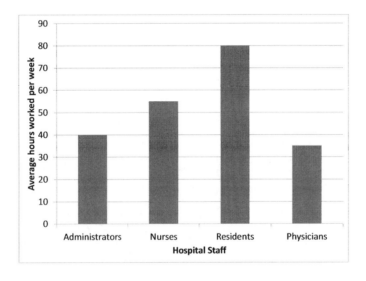

a. The dependent variable is Nurses. The independent variable is Physicians.
b. The dependent variable is Physicians. The independent variable is Nurses.
c. The dependent variable is Hospital Staff. The independent variable is Average hours worked per week.
d. The dependent variable is Average hours worked per week. The independent variable is Hospital Staff.

27. How many milligrams are in 5 grams?
a. 5 g = 0.005 mg
b. 5 g = 50 mg
c. 5 g = 500 mg
d. 5 g = 5000 mg

28. About how much does an apple weigh?
   a. 1 mg
   b. 0.001 g
   c. 100 g
   d. 1000 kg

29. Which unit of measure would be used to describe the length of a bone?
   a. grams
   b. liters
   c. meters
   d. pounds

30. Use the figure below to determine the distance between marks 1 and 4. The marks are evenly spaced two centimeters apart.

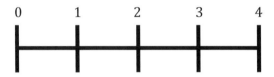

   a. 2 cm
   b. 6 cm
   c. 8 cm
   d. 10 cm

31. Two even integers and one odd integer are multiplied together. Which of the following could be their product?
   a. 3.75
   b. 9
   c. 16.2
   d. 24

32. There are $\frac{80\ mg}{0.8\ ml}$ in Acetaminophen Concentrated Infant Drops. If the proper dosage for a four year old child is 240 mg, how many milliliters should the child receive?
   a. 0.8 ml
   b. 1.6 ml
   c. 2.4 ml
   d. 3.2 ml

33. Using the chart below, which equation describes the relationship between x and y?

   a. $x = 3y$
   b. $y = 3x$
   c. $y = \frac{1}{3}x$
   d. $\frac{x}{y} = 3$

x	y
2	6
3	9
4	12
5	15

34. On a highway map, the scale indicates that 1 inch represents 45 miles. If the distance on the map is 3.2 inches, how far is the actual distance?
    a. 45 miles
    b. 54 miles
    c. 112 miles
    d. 144 miles

Section 3. Science	Number of Questions: **54**
	Time Limit: **66 Minutes**

1. Which item below is part of the circulatory system?
   a. Kidneys
   b. Lungs
   c. Heart
   d. Stomach

2. Which item below is NOT part of the digestive system?
   a. Stomach
   b. Brain
   c. Mouth
   d. Esophagus

3. Which item below best describes the primary function of the nervous system?
   a. The nervous system is the center of communication in the body.
   b. The nervous system is primarily responsible for helping the body breathe.
   c. The nervous system transports blood throughout the body.
   d. The nervous system helps the body break down food.

4. Which of the following systems is primarily responsible for helping the body breathe?
   a. Nervous system
   b. Circulatory system
   c. Digestive system
   d. Respiratory system

5. Which system helps fight illness?
   a. Immune system
   b. Digestive system
   c. Nervous system
   d. Urinary system

6. Which item in the following list is NOT one of the major types of bones in the human body?
   a. Dense bone
   b. Long bone
   c. Short bone
   d. Irregular bone

7. Which of the following bone types is embedded in tendons?
   a. Long bones
   b. Sesamoid bones
   c. Flat bones
   d. Vertical bones

8. Which of the following factors could cause population growth in the United States?
   a. Fatal disease
   b. Migration from the United States to Europe
   c. Increased birth rate
   d. Increased death rate

9. Which of the following does NOT affect fertility in women?
   a. Smoking
   b. Stress
   c. Alcohol consumption
   d. All the above factors affect fertility in women.

10. If scientists created a cure for cancer, how would the population most likely be affected?
    a. The population would decrease.
    b. The population would increase.
    c. The population would remain the same.
    d. The population would end.

11. Each year, 3% of the people in country Q move to a different country. However, 1% of the people move back the next year. How is the population of country Q most likely affected by this movement of its citizens?
    a. The population decreases.
    b. The population increases.
    c. The population remains unchanged.
    d. The population is overcrowded.

12. Which of the following scenarios best illustrates the process of natural selection?
    a. When food was no longer available on the ground, the giraffes with long necks were able to eat leaves from tall trees. These giraffes survived and reproduced, creating more giraffes with long necks. After some time, all giraffes had long necks.
    b. When food was no longer available on the ground, the giraffes looked to other animals to give them food each day.
    c. When food was no longer available on the ground, the giraffes wondered how they would eat.
    d. When food was no longer available on the ground, the giraffes became extinct.

13. The term "*Homo sapiens*" belongs to which two categories of the biological classification?
    a. *Homo* is the kingdom and *sapiens* designates the phylum.
    b. *Homo* is the phylum and sapiens designates the kingdom.
    c. Homo is the species and sapiens designates the genus.
    d. Homo is the genus and *sapiens* designates the species.

14. Which part of the cell is often called the cell "power house" because it provides energy for cellular functions?
    a. Nucleus
    b. Cell membrane
    c. Mitochondria
    d. Cytoplasm

15. What function do ribosomes serve within the cell?
    a. Ribosomes are responsible for cell movement.
    b. Ribosomes aid in protein synthesis.
    c. Ribosomes help protect the cell from its environment.
    d. Ribosomes have enzymes that help with digestion.

16. What is the most likely reason that cells differentiate?
    a. Cells differentiate to avoid looking like all the cells around them.
    b. Cells differentiate so that simple, non-specialized cells can become highly specialized cells.
    c. Cells differentiate so that multicellular organisms will remain the same size.
    d. Cells differentiate for no apparent reason.

17. How is meiosis similar to mitosis?
    a. Both produce daughter cells that are genetically identical.
    b. Both produce daughter cells that are genetically different.
    c. Both occur in humans, other animals, and plants.
    d. Both occur asexually.

18. Which of the following statements is TRUE about photosynthesis and respiration?
    a. Photosynthesis occurs in both plants and animals.
    b. Respiration occurs in both plants and animals.
    c. Photosynthesis occurs only in animals, while respiration occurs only in plants.
    d. Photosynthesis occurs only in plants, while respiration occurs only in animals.

19. How do DNA and RNA function together as part of the human genome?
    a. DNA carries genetic information from RNA to the cell cytoplasm.
    b. RNA carries genetic information from DNA to the cell cytoplasm.
    c. DNA and RNA carry genetic information from the cell nucleus to the cytoplasm.
    d. DNA and RNA do not interact within the cell.

20. Which statement below best describes genetic mutations?
     a. Genetic mutations are changes in DNA that occur systematically at fast rates.
     b. Genetic mutations are changes in DNA that occur spontaneously at low rates.
     c. Genetic mutations occur when DNA remains the same over relatively short time intervals.
     d. Genetic mutations occur when DNA remains the same over relatively long time intervals.

21. What process should the DNA within a cell undergo before cell replication?
     a. The DNA should quadruple so that daughter cells have more than enough DNA material after cell division.
     b. The DNA should triple so that daughter cells have three times the amount of DNA material after cell division.
     c. The DNA should replicate so that daughter cells have the same amount of DNA material after cell division.
     d. The DNA should split so that daughter cells have half the amount of DNA material after cell division.

22. What basic molecular unit enables hereditary information to be transmitted from parent to offspring?
     a. genes
     b. blood
     c. organs
     d. hair

23. Which statement most accurately compares and contrasts the structures of DNA and RNA?
     a. Both DNA and RNA have 4 nucleotide bases. Three of the bases are the same but the fourth base is thymine in DNA and uracil in RNA.
     b. Both DNA and RNA have the same 4 nucleotide bases. However, the nucleotides bond differently in the DNA when compared to RNA.
     c. Both DNA and RNA have 6 nucleotide bases. However, the shape of DNA is a triple helix and the shape of RNA is a double helix.
     d. Both DNA and RNA have a double helix structure. However, DNA contains 6 nucleotide bases and RNA contains 4 nucleotide bases.

24. Which of the following characteristics is part of a person's genotype?
     a. Brown eyes that appear hazel in the sunlight
     b. CFTR genes that causes cystic fibrosis
     c. Black hair that grows rapidly
     d. Being a fast runner

Let *B* represent the dominant gene for a full head of hair, and let *b* represent the recessive gene for male pattern baldness. The following Punnett square represents the offspring of two people with recessive genes for baldness.

	B	b
B	Possibility 1	Possibility 2
b	Possibility 3	Possibility 4

The next two questions are based on the above information.

25. According to the Punnett square, which possibility would produce an offspring with male pattern baldness?
   a. Possibility 1
   b. Possibility 2
   c. Possibility 3
   d. Possibility 4

26. According to the Punnett square, which possibility would produce an offspring with a full head of hair?
   a. Possibility 1
   b. Possibility 2
   c. Possibility 3
   d. All of the above.

27. Which of the following celestial bodies serves as a major external source of heat, light, and energy for Earth?
   a. Mars
   b. The Big Dipper
   c. The sun
   d. The moon

28. Which of the following reactions is an example of oxidation?
   a. Copper loses 2 electrons.
   b. Copper gains 2 electrons.
   c. Copper loses 2 neutrons.
   d. Copper gains 2 neutrons.

29. Chemical C is a catalyst in the reaction between chemical A and chemical B. What is the effect of chemical C?
   a. Chemical C increases the rate of the reaction between A and B.
   b. Chemical C decreases the rate of the reaction between A and B.
   c. Chemical C converts A from an acid to a base.
   d. Chemical C converts A from a base to an acid.

30. What type of molecules are enzymes?
    a. Water molecules
    b. Protein molecules
    c. Tripolar molecules
    d. Inorganic molecules

31. Fill in the blanks in this sentence: Acids have a pH that is _____ while bases have a pH that is

___.
    a. Acids have a pH that is <u>less than 7</u> while bases have a pH that is <u>equal to 7</u>.
    b. Acids have a pH that is equal to 7 while bases have a pH that is greater than 7.
    c. Acids have a pH that is less than 7 while bases have a pH that is greater than 7.
    d. Acids have a pH that is <u>greater than 7</u> while bases have a pH that is <u>less than 7</u>.

32. What type of chemical bond connects the sodium and chlorine atoms in a molecule of salt?
    a. Ionic bond
    b. Covalent bond
    c. Coordinated bond
    d. Salty bond

33. Which of the following statements is NOT a chemical property of water?
    a. Water molecules contain hydrogen and oxygen atoms.
    b. Water has a pH of 7.
    c. Water molecules have covalent bonds.
    d. Water molecules have ionic bonds.

34. Consider the following statements about a ball. Which of these statements describes the ball possessing the most kinetic energy?
    a. A ball is sitting on top of a hill.
    b. A ball is rolling down a hill.
    c. A ball is resting in a bucket.
    d. A ball is being held in someone's hand.

35. An atom has 5 protons, 5 neutrons, and 6 electrons. What is the electric charge of this atom?
    a. Neutral
    b. Positive
    c. Negative
    d. Undetermined

36. Which of the following statements most accurately describes the major components of an atom?
    a. Positrons and negatrons are located in the atomic nucleus while neutrons orbit the nucleus.
    b. Positrons and neutrons are located in the atomic nucleus while negatrons orbit the nucleus.
    c. Protons and electrons are located in the atomic nucleus while neutrons orbit the nucleus.
    d. Protons and neutrons are located in the atomic nucleus while electrons orbit the nucleus.

37. What type of chemical bond is formed when electrons are shared between atoms?
    a. Covalent bond
    b. Ionic bond
    c. Dipolar bond
    d. Molecular bond

38. The table below contains information from the periodic table of elements.

Element	Atomic number	Approximate atomic weight
H	1	1
He	2	4
Li	3	7
Be	4	9

Which pattern below best describes the elements listed in the table?
    a. The elements are arranged in order by weight with H being the heaviest atom and Be being the lightest atom.
    b. The elements are arranged in order by electron charge with H having the most electrons and Be having the fewest electrons.
    c. The elements are arranged in order by protons with H having the most protons and Be having the fewest protons.
    d. The elements are arranged in order by protons with H having the fewest protons and Be having the most protons.

39. Which statement best describes the difference between a liquid and a solid?
    a. Atoms in a liquid have a fixed structure, but solids maintain the shape of their container.
    b. Liquids maintain the shape of their container, but atoms in a solid have a fixed structure.
    c. Atoms in a solid flow easily, but atoms in a liquid do not flow.
    d. Solids and liquids are made of different kinds of atoms.

40. The process of changing from a liquid to a gas is called _____?
    a. Freezing
    b. Condensation
    c. Vaporization
    d. Sublimation

41. A nurse wants to investigate how different environmental factors affect her patients' body temperatures. Which tool would be the most helpful when the nurse conducts her investigation?
    a. Scale
    b. Yard stick
    c. Thermometer
    d. Blood pressure monitor

42. A scientific study has over 2000 data points. Which of the following methods is most likely to help the researcher gain usable information from the data?
    a. Use statistical analysis to understand trends in the data.
    b. Look at each individual data point, and try to create a trend.
    c. Eliminate 90% of the data so that the sample size is more manageable.
    d. Stare at the data until a pattern pops out.

43. Many years ago, people believed that flies were created from spoiled food because spoiled food that was left out in the open often contained fly larvae. So a scientist placed fresh food in a sealed container for an extended period of time. The food spoiled, but no fly larvae were found in the food that was sealed. Based on this evidence, what is the most likely reason that spoiled food left out in the open often contained fly larvae?
    a. The spoiled food evolved into fly larvae.
    b. Since the food was left out in the open, flies would lay eggs in the food.
    c. Fly larvae were spontaneously generated by the spoiled food.
    d. People only imagined they saw fly larvae in the spoiled food.

44. The average life expectancy in the 21st century is about 75 years. The average life expectancy in the 19th century was about 40 years. What is a possible explanation for the longer life expectancy in the present age?
    a. Advances in medical technology enable people to live longer.
    b. Knowledge about how basic cleanliness can help avoid illness has enabled people to live longer.
    c. The creation of various vaccines has enabled people to live longer.
    d. All of the statements above offer reasonable explanations for longer life expectancy.

45. A doctor needs to convince his boss to approve a test for a patient. Which statement below best communicates a scientific argument that justifies the need for the test?
    a. The patient looks like he needs this test.
    b. The doctor feels that the patient needs this test.
    c. The patient's symptoms and health history suggest that this test will enable the correct diagnosis to help the patient.
    d. The patient has excellent insurance that will pay for several tests, and the doctor would like to run as many tests as possible.

46. A hospital board wants to investigate how long people wait to see a doctor when visiting the emergency room (ER). Which statement provides the best reason to conduct this investigation?
    a. The board can use ER wait times to help themselves feel good.
    b. The board can use ER wait times to determine if the ER is understaffed.
    c. The board can use ER wait times for advertising purposes.
    d. There is no sound reason to conduct this investigation.

47. Which of the following statements provides the best reason to include technology in scientific research?

  a. Technology can provide the ability to efficiently and effectively collect and analyze an extremely large amount of data.

  b. Technology can be used to create nice pictures of the research results.

  c. Technology can help researchers spend more time with their families.

  d. Technology should not be included in scientific research.

48. Which of the following statements is NOT a reason to include mathematics in scientific research?

  a. Researchers can use mathematics to sway research outcomes in whatever direction they choose.

  b. Statistical mathematics can help researchers discover patterns and trends in large amounts of data.

  c. Mathematics enables data analysis to be objective instead of subjective.

  d. Researchers can use mathematics to help define measurable research goals.

49. Which of the following structures has the lowest blood pressure?

  a. arteries

  b. arteriole

  c. venule

  d. vein

50. Which of the heart chambers is the most muscular?

  a. left atrium

  b. right atrium

  c. left ventricle

  d. right ventricle

51. Which part of the brain interprets sensory information?

  a. cerebrum

  b. hindbrain

  C cerebellum

  d. medulla oblongata

52. Which of the following proteins is produced by cartilage?

  a. actin

  b. estrogen

  c. collagen

  d. myosin

53. Which component of the nervous system is responsible for lowering the heart rate?
    a. central nervous system
    b. sympathetic nervous system
    c. parasympathetic nervous system
    d. distal nervous system

54. How much air does an adult inhale in an average breath?
    a. 500 mL
    b. 750 mL
    c. 1000 mL
    d. 1250 mL

Section 4. English and Language Usage	Number of Questions: **34**
	Time Limit: **34 Minutes**

1. Which of the following sentences shows the correct way to separate the items in the series?
    a. These are actual cities in the United States: Unalaska, Alaska; Yreka, California; Two Egg, Florida; and Boring, Maryland.
    b. These are actual cities in the United States: Unalaska; Alaska, Yreka; California, Two Egg; Florid, and Boring; Maryland.
    c. These are actual cities in the United States: Unalaska, Alaska, Yreka, California, Two Egg, Florida, and Boring, Maryland.
    d. These are actual cities in the United States: Unalaska Alaska, Yreka California, Two Egg Florida, and Boring Maryland.

2. Adella knows how high the stakes are in her trading job at the investment bank, so she is very _____ about following the rules and fulfilling all of the requirements. Which of the following words should be placed in the blank?
    a. conscientous
    b. consientious
    c. conscientious
    d. consciencious

3. _____ going on vacation to _____ house on Lake Chelan, and they plan to water ski and parasail while _____. Which of the following sets of words would correctly complete the sentence?
    a. Their; there; they're
    b. They're; their; there
    c. They're; there; their
    d. There; they're; their

4. Which of the following sentences demonstrates the correct use of an apostrophe?
    a. Lyle works for the courthouse, and among his responsibilities is getting the jurors meal's.
    b. Lyle works for the courthouse, and among his responsibilities is getting the juror's meals.
    c. Lyle works for the courthouse, and among his responsibilities is getting the jurors' meals.
    d. Lyle works for the courthouse, and among his responsibilities is getting the jurors meals'.

5. Which of the following is a complex sentence?
    a. Milton's favorite meal is spaghetti and meatballs, along with a side salad and garlic toast.
    b. Before Ernestine purchases a book, she always checks to see if the library has it.
    c. Desiree prefers warm, sunny weather, but her twin sister Destiny likes a crisp, cold day.
    d. Ethel, Ben, and Alice are working together on a school project about deteriorating dams.

6. Finlay flatly refused to take part in the piano recital, so his parents had to *cajole* him with the promise of a trip to his favorite toy store. Which of the following is the best definition of *cajole* as it is used in the sentence above?
   a. prevent
   b. threaten
   c. insist
   d. coax

7. Which of the following nouns is the correct plural form of the word *tempo*?
   a. tempo
   b. tempae
   c. tempi
   d. tempos

8. Which of the following sentences follows the rules of capitalization?
   a. Kristia knows that her Aunt Jo will be visiting, but she is not sure if her uncle will be there as well.
   b. During a visit to the monastery, Jess interviewed brother Mark about the daily prayer schedule.
   c. Leah spoke to cousin Martha about her summer plans to drive from Colorado to Arizona.
   d. Justinia will be staying with family in the outer banks during the early Fall.

9. To register a vehicle, each person will need ____ proof of insurance, proof of a passed safety inspection, and a completed registration application.
Which of the following choices best completes the sentence above?
   a. their
   b. its
   c. the
   d. his or her

10. Which of the following sentences does not use correct punctuation to separate independent clauses?
   a. Anne likes to add salsa to her scrambled eggs; Gordon unaccountably likes his with peanut butter.
   b. Anne likes to add salsa to her scrambled eggs, however Gordon unaccountably likes his with peanut butter.
   c. Anne likes to add salsa to her scrambled eggs. Gordon unaccountably likes his with peanut butter.
   d. Anne likes to add salsa to her scrambled eggs, but Gordon unaccountably likes his with peanut butter.

11. Fenella wanted to attend the concert. She also wanted to attend the reception at the art gallery. She tried to find a way to do both in one evening. She failed. Which of the following options best combines the sentences above? Consider both style and clarity when choosing a response.
    a. Although Fenella wanted to attend the concert, she also wanted to attend the reception at the art gallery, so she tried to find a way to do both in one evening. She failed.
    b. Fenella wanted to attend both the concert and the reception at the art gallery, but she failed to find a way to do both in one evening.
    c. Fenella failed to find a way to attend both the concert and the reception at the art gallery.
    d. Because Fenella wanted to attend both the concert and the reception at the art gallery, she tried to find a way to do both in one evening. Unfortunately, she failed.

12. Which of the following nouns is the correct plural form of the word *human*?
    a. humans
    b. humen
    c. human's
    d. humans'

13. The word *permeate*, meaning "to penetrate or pervade," is made up of two parts with a Latin origin: the root *meare*, which means "to pass," and the prefix *per-*. Based on the current definition of the word *permeate*, which of the following is the most likely meaning of the prefix *per-*?
    a. across
    b. by
    c. with
    d. through

14. The following words share a common Greek-based suffix: *anthropology, cosmetology, etymology,* and *genealogy*. What is the most likely meaning of the suffix *-logy*?
    a. record
    b. study
    c. affinity
    d. fear

15. Jacob had been worried about the speech, but in the end he did well. Which of the following words functions as an adverb in the sentence?
    a. worried
    b. about
    c. but
    d. well

16. Most doctors ____ that there ____ a lot of reasons to add a daily multivitamin to the diet. Which of the following sets of words correctly completes the sentence?
    a. agree; is
    b. agree; are
    c. agrees; is
    d. agrees; are

3 TEAS Practice Tests by Exam Review Press

17. Which of the following sentences contains a correct example of subject-verb agreement?
     a. Neither Jeanne nor Pauline like the dinner options on the menu.
     b. All of the council likes the compromise that they have reached about property taxes.
     c. The faculty of the math department were unable to agree on the curriculum changes.
     d. Both Clara and Don feels that they need to be more proactive in checking on the contractors.

18. The guest speaker was undoubtedly an *erudite* scholar, but his comments on nomological determinism seemed to go over the heads of the students in the audience. Which of the following best explains the meaning of *erudite* in the sentence?
     a. authentic
     b. arrogant
     c. faulty
     d. knowledgeable

19. Wearing white to a funeral is considered by many to be _____. Which of the following correctly completes the sentence?
     a. sacrelegious
     b. sacriligious
     c. sacrilegious
     d. sacreligious

20. Which of the following demonstrates the correct use of a hyphen?
     a. super-sede
     b. cross-word
     c. self-evident
     d. semi-final

21. Due to concerns about overspending, the city council conducted an investigation into the budget and then facilitated a discourse among local residents about ways to cut spending. Which of the following best removes the nominalization from the sentence?
     a. Due to concerns about overspending, the city council facilitated a discourse among local residents after conducting an investigation into the budget.
     b. Concerned about overspending, the city council investigated the budget and then discussed ways to cut spending with residents.
     c. Concerned about overspending, the city council investigated the budget and then opened the floor up to local residents about ways to cut spending.
     d. Due to concerns about overspending, the city council reviewed the budget and then turned over the decision about ways to cut spending to residents.

22. Which of the following is a simple sentence?
     a. Ben likes baseball, but Joseph likes basketball.
     b. It looks like rain; be sure to bring an umbrella.
     c. Although he was tired, Edgar still attended the recital.
     d. Marjorie and Thomas planned an exciting trip to Maui.

23. Anne-Charlotte and I will be driving together to the picnic this weekend. Which of the following words functions as a pronoun in the sentence?
    a. be
    b. this
    c. together
    d. I

24. Which of the following demonstrates the correct use of quotation marks?
    a. The professor read aloud from the first chapter of David Copperfield, entitled "I am Born."
    b. The professor read aloud from the first chapter of "David Copperfield," entitled I am Born.
    c. The professor read aloud from the first chapter of David Copperfield, entitled 'I am Born.'
    d. The professor read aloud from the first chapter of "David Copperfield," entitled 'I am Born.'

25. Which of the following sentences is the best in terms of style, clarity, and conciseness?
    a. Ava has a leap year birthday; she is really twenty, and her friends like to joke that she is only five years old.
    b. Because Ava has a leap year birthday, her friends like to joke that she is only five years old when she is really twenty.
    c. Ava is twenty years old, her friends like to joke that she is five because she has a leap year birthday.
    d. Although Ava has a leap year birthday, she is twenty years old, but her friends like to joke that she is five.

26. The housekeeper Mrs. Vanderbroek had a fixed daily routine for running the manor, and was not particularly *amenable* to any suggested changes. Which of the following best explains the meaning of *amenable* as it is used in the sentence?
    a. capable
    b. agreeable
    c. obstinate
    d. critical

27. A quick review of all available housing options indicated that Casper had little choice but to rent for now and wait for a better time to buy. Which of the following words does not function as an adjective in the sentence?
    a. quick
    b. available
    c. little
    d. rent

28. Roan and ____ were so angry about the gag gift that they refused to speak to Elsie and ____ for two months.
    a. she; I
    b. she; me
    c. her; I
    d. her; me

29. Tamara had a problem with her furnace. She checked the phonebook for repair shops. She called two different repair shops. They were closest to her home. The first quoted a very high price. The second quoted a more reasonable price. Which of the following options best combines the sentences above? Consider style, clarity, and conciseness when selecting your response.

    a. Tamara had a problem with her furnace, so she checked the phonebook for repair shops. She called two different shops that were closest to her home. Although the first quoted a very high price, the second quoted a more reasonable price.

    b. After discovering that she had a problem with her furnace, Tamara checked the phone book for repair shops and called two different shops. These two were closest to her home. It turned out that the first quoted a very high price, but the second was more reasonable.

    c. Of the two furnace repair shops that Tamara called, the first quoted a very high price, but the second quoted a more reasonable price. Tamara needed to have her furnace repaired after discovering that there was a problem with it.

    d. When Tamara had a problem with her furnace, she checked the phonebook for repair shops that were closest to her home and called two different shops. The first quoted a very high price, but the second was more reasonable.

30. The Constitution mentions the right to _____ arms, but one common mistake is to spell this as though the Founding Fathers were ensuring the right to go sleeveless. Which of the following words correctly completes the sentence?

    a. bear
    b. bare
    c. barre
    d. baire

31. Which word is *not* used correctly in the context of the following sentence?
There is no real distinction among the two treatment protocols recommended online.

    a. real
    b. among
    c. protocols
    d. online

Choose the meaning of the underlined words in the sentences below.

32. Her concern for him was **<u>sincere.</u>**
    a. intense
    b. genuine
    c. brief
    d. misunderstood

33. He is a very **<u>courteous</u>** young man.
    a. handsome
    b. polite
    c. inconsiderate
    d. odd

34. Spanish is a difficult language to **comprehend**.
    a. learn
    b. speak
    c. understand
    d. appreciate

Answer Explanations

Reading Answer Explanations

1. B: The word *intermittent* suggests that something occurs at imprecise intervals, so answer choice B is the best synonym. Answer choices A and D suggest the exact opposite of the meaning indicated in the sentence. Answer choice C likely reflects another element of the woman's labor, but it has nothing to do with the meaning of the word *intermittent*.

2. B: The context of the sentence suggests that Edith is emphasizing the temperature of the plate. In this sentence, dialogue is conveyed with the quotation marks, and part of the quotation is not in a bold font. The bold font must mean something other than dialogue, so answer choice A cannot be correct. The sentence clearly indicates that Edith speaks to the man, so answer choice C makes little sense. Additionally, there is no reason to believe that Edith is angry. Rather, she is concerned about the man's safety. Therefore, answer choice D is incorrect.

3. D: In this sentence, the information in parentheses appears to be examples of humanities disciplines. (Additionally, the abbreviation "e.g." stands for the Latin phrase *exempli gratia*, meaning "for example.") Thus, answer choice D is the correct option. There is no reason to believe that the information in parentheses is either an error or a correction, so answer choices A and C are incorrect. While answer choice C has promise – suggesting that the information in parentheses is an addition to information already provided – it is not as strong as option D, since option D provides the more logical explanation about the parenthetical details being examples.

4. C: Only the word *neglect* can fall between the guide words *needs* and *negotiate* on a dictionary page. The words *needle* and *nectar* would come before *needs*, and the word *neigh* would follow *negotiate*.

5. D: The chapter title refers to the *fictional* words of Dorothy L. Sayers, and letters generally do not fall under the category of fiction. Novels, plays, and mysteries, however, usually do.

6. C: An expository passage seeks to *expose* information by explaining or defining it in detail. As this passage focuses on describing the written works of Dorothy L. Sayers, it may safely be considered expository. The author is not necessarily telling a story, something one might expect from a strictly narrative passage. (Additionally, the author's main point, that of explaining why Sayers was such a versatile writer, represents a kind of thesis statement for shaping the overall focus of the passage. A narrative passage would focus more on simply telling the story of Sayers's life.) At no point is the author attempting to persuade the reader about anything, and there is nothing particularly technical about the passage. Rather, it is a focused look at Sayers's educational background and how she developed into a writer of many genres; this makes it solidly expository.

7. A: As indicated in the answer explanation above, the main focus of the passage is Sayers's versatility as a writer. The first paragraph notes this and then begins discussing her education, introducing the experience that would inform her later accomplishments. The second paragraph then follows this up with specifics about the types of writing she did. Answer choice B would be correct if the passage were more narrative than expository. Answer choices C and D focus on specific publications for which Sayers is remembered, but both are too limited to be considered a representative summary of the entire passage.

8. B: The mention of an "unexpectedly good education" represents an opinion on the part of the author. As the author does not follow this up with an explanation about *why* such an education would be unexpectedly good, the statement is simply a moment of bias on the author's part, rather than an element within the larger argument. There is no bias in the other answer choices. Answer choices A and C are factual statements about Sayers's life and work. Answer choice D, while it might hint vaguely at disapproval on the author's part (who might, perhaps, wish to know Sayers's reasons), is not necessarily a statement containing bias. It is indeed true that Sayers turned down the doctorate of divinity, and it is also true that her reasons for doing so are unknown. Only answer choice B conveys an opinion of the author.

9. D: A search for early maps by one of the first people to study geography would certainly take Jorgen to the 900 section of the library: History, geography, and biography. For this particular study, there is no reason for Jorgen to look among books on philosophy and psychology, social sciences, or technical and applied science.

10. D: The sieve of Eratosthenes is a mathematical tool, so Jorgen should go to the science and mathematics section. While the sieve might be used in certain computer applications, there is no specific indication of this. As a result, answer choice D is a better option than answer choice A. Also, Jorgen has no reason to check the philosophy and psychology or languages sections to find out more about a mathematical topic.

11. B: Section 400 is the section on languages, so it is a good place to look for more information about the letters of the Greek alphabet. Jorgen would be unlikely to find anything useful in the sections on religion; arts and recreation; or history, geography, and biography. (It is arguable, of course, that the use of Greek letters in relation to Christianity – Christ as the "alpha" and the "omega," or the beginning and the end – make the religion section a possible place to look for the meaning of "beta." But, this is certainly not the first place Jorgen should look, as the information would be buried in a book about Christianity. Checking for a Greek language guide would be far quicker.)

12. D: Section 800 features works of literature, so that is the best place for Jorgen to begin looking for *The Iliad* and *The Odyssey*. The philosophy and psychology section will likely contain references to these works, but Jorgen would still have to go to the literature section to obtain the works themselves. The same thing can be said about the religion and arts and recreation sections.

13. C: While planning her daughter's wedding, Marci is likely to find picking out a paint color for the living room *unimportant*. Therefore, answer choice C is the most logical option. Choosing a paint color might also be meaningless at the moment, but it is not without meaning altogether. It is simply not as important. Answer choice A infers more than the sentence implies. Answer choice B could be forced into the sentence (if Marci was looking for a distraction from the stress of wedding planning, for instance), but it is not natural, and it is certainly not a synonym for *peripheral*. Answer choice D makes little sense in the context of the sentence.

14. B: Latvia's total population was around two million in 2011. Twenty-five percent of this number is about 500,000 people. The Russian population is closest to this number. The chart indicates that the Latvian population was around 1,300,000 in 2011; the Ukrainian population was well under 200,000; the German population was even lower than the Ukrainian population.

15. D: According to the chart, the Latvian and German populations are the only ones that decreased. In terms of sheer numbers, the Latvian population decrease exceeded the German population decrease by around 2,000 people. But in terms of percentage, which is what the question asks about, the German population decrease is far greater. An ethnic group that declines from around 70,000 people to just over 3,000 people has decreased by over 90 percent. The Latvian population, on the other hand, decreased by only about five percent.

16. B: The Russian population of Latvia decreased the most since 1991. The Latvian population decreased slightly, but not to the same degree. The Ukrainian population decreased by an even smaller percentage since 1991. The German population remained relatively unchanged between 1991 and 2011.

17. C: On the chart, the only ethnic group that represents approximately one percent of the population after World War II and approximately three percent by 1991 is the Ukrainian population. The Latvian and Russian populations represent much larger percentages of the total population of Latvia. The German population decreased significantly during this time period.

18. C: As the final step indicates, the new word should end in Y. This immediately eliminates answer choice D. Answer choice A adds an L when a second one is not required, and answer choice B adds two Ts to a word that has none. Only answer choice C follows all of the directions to spell the new word: REPLAY.

19. A: Klara's success is clearly the result of diligence, so answer choice A must be correct. It is possible that her diligence was also silent, but the sentence does not indicate this. Answer choice B, then, cannot be correct. A moderate commitment by an average student would not lead to exemplary results, so answer choice C is incorrect. Answer choice D makes no sense in the context of the sentence.

20. D: Puffed rice is a dry breakfast cereal, and therefore contains (or might contain) a dairy product. Breaded chicken parmesan contains both bread crumbs and parmesan cheese; the cheese is certainly a dairy product, and bread crumbs are on the warning list from the doctor. A sliced turkey sandwich contains deli meat and bread, both of which are discouraged by Flemming's doctor. Yogurt made from coconut milk, however, is meant to be a dairy-free alternative, so it should be a safe choice for Flemming.

21. C: Chapter III of the manual contains information about adjusting the climate within the vehicle, so it is here that Regina will find the instructions she needs to adjust the air conditioning. Chapter I would be the best choice if the manual did *not* also include Chapter III. The chapter on safety options would probably not contain information about how to operate the air conditioning, so answer choice B is incorrect. Regina should definitely adjust the air conditioning before she begins driving, but the information needed to do this is not likely to be found in Chapter IV.

22. B: Chapter V discusses routine maintenance, and oil changes fall firmly in this category. With this chapter available, there is no reason for Regina to check the chapters on pre-driving and driving, emergencies, or consumer resources.

23. D: A list of dealerships is most likely to be found in the section on consumer resources. With this chapter available, there is no reason for Regina to check the chapters on vehicle instruments; audio, climate, and voice controls; or routine maintenance.

24. D: An overheating vehicle is definitely an emergency, so Regina would need to consult Chapter VI. The other chapters contain useful information that Regina will need once her vehicle is back in working order, but until then she should focus on the information in the chapter about emergency situations.

25. B: As most students discover, Wikipedia is not considered a reliable source or a particularly scholarly one. The Encyclopedia Britannica is, however, as are Science.gov (which would contain officially recognized information provided by a government organization) and LexisNexis (a reputable site containing legal and educational resources).

26. C: The word *temperate* can have a number of meanings, including "modest" and "conservative." In the context of the poem, however, the best meaning is "agreeable," because the poet is clearly saying that his beloved is lovelier and more agreeable than a summer day. The meaning of "immoderate" is the opposite of that suggested by the word *temperate* in the poem.

27. C: The slash between the sentences indicates the break in the lines of poetry. The reader knows this is a poem, because question 26 refers to the lines as part of a sonnet. The most obvious reason to separate the sentences would be to note where the poet has divided the lines. There is not enough of the sonnet to suggest that the slash indicates different stanzas. (In addition, a Shakespearean sonnet does not typically have stanzas as they are most often recognized in poetry.) The question mark on its own indicates a question; the slash is not needed to indicate this, or to indicate that the statement that follows is a direct answer to the question. Similarly, the end punctuation indicates the end of each sentence. A slash is not necessary for this. (Otherwise, there would be a slash at the end of both sentences, instead of one between the two.)

28. D: Eczema is a topical condition, so Chapter 12 (section D) would be the most appropriate place to look. Eczema is not specific to either men or women, nor is it specific to adults, so Chapter 8 would not be the best place to look. Finally, eczema is neither a respiratory condition nor a digestive condition.

29. A: This question asks the reader to consider the distinction between a recognized respiratory condition (Chapter 10) and a children's condition (Chapter 7). In this case, the first and best place to check is Chapter 7, because it addresses conditions specific to children, and it describes herbs that may be useful in treating these conditions. Herbs, like pharmaceuticals, need to be used carefully, and the type of herbal remedy that would be used to treat an adult respiratory condition is not necessarily the same one that would be used to treat a respiratory condition in a child. Additionally, the dosage would certainly be different, so the chapter on children's conditions is the correct place to look. Chapters 9 and 12 (immunity and detox, respectively) would not contain useful information for this particular situation.

30. C: Chapter 5 contains information about using herbs in beverages. Since Clothilde is looking for ways to use the elderflower to make tea and wine, this chapter should be useful. Chapter 3 would not likely contain information that would be useful in this situation. Chapter 4 discusses using herbs in food, so Clothilde is unlikely to find anything in this section about beverages. Chapter 13 would certainly be the place to look in the index of herbs, but this chapter would most likely contain a listing of the herb and a summary of its properties, rather than recommendations for how to use it in tea or wine making.

31. B: Chapter 3 contains information about caring for herbs, so it is the first place Clothilde should look. The herb is clearly already planted, so Chapter 2 will not be of much use in this case. Again, Chapter 13 would certainly be the place to look in the index of herbs, but this chapter would most likely contain a listing of the herb and a summary of its properties, rather than recommendations for maintaining the plant. Chapter 14, the alphabetical listing for herbs J-O, is unlikely to contain any information either about caring for herbs in general or about the elderberry in particular.

32. C: Only Cosette fulfills all of the clearly stated requirements in the ad. She does not smoke (and is, in fact, allergic to cigarette smoke), and she needs a quiet place to study in a house that is advertised as having quiet occupants. Also implied is Cosette's need to be close to the university, since she is likely going to be studying for classes. Frances has a dog, and this is not allowed according to the ad. Adelaide is looking for a short-term lease, and the other occupants prefer a long-term renter. Felix is male, and the other occupants are looking for a female renter.

33. B: Sculpture is not typically classified as a performing art.

34. B: For two pounds of each type of tea, Wholesale Tea's price would be $96, which is the best price. Tea Heaven's price would be $102. Tea by The Pound's price would be $104. Tea Express's price would be the same as Tea Heaven's price: $102.

35. B: Wholesale Tea would have the best price for these specific blends. The price for one pound of Earl Grey and two pounds of green tea would be $78. Tea Heaven's price would be $87. Tea by The Pound's price would be $83. Tea Express's price would be $88.

36. D: Kiev is the capital of Ukraine, which is not part of Northern Europe according to the information provided in the question. (It is not one of the Scandinavian countries, it is not one of the Baltic states, and it is certainly not part of Great Britain.) Copenhagen is the capital of Denmark, and Oslo is the capital of Norway. Both of these regions are part of Scandinavia. London is the capital of England in Great Britain.

37. A: Portugal is the other country on the Iberian Peninsula. It is unique among countries in Southern Europe because it does not have a coastline along the Mediterranean Sea or the Black Sea. The western and southern coasts of Portugal border the Atlantic Ocean. Italy and Cyprus are not on the Iberian Peninsula, and both have Mediterranean coasts. Bulgaria is also not on the Iberian Peninsula, and its eastern coast borders the Black Sea.

38. C: The only logical conclusion that can be made based on the announcement is that the library has applied a fee to Internet usage beyond 30 minutes to discourage patrons from spending too long on the computers. There is nothing in the announcement to suggest that the library plans to add more computers. The announcement mentions a limited number of computers, but there is no indication that there are plans to change this fact. The announcement makes no mention of the library's budget, so it is impossible to infer that the library is facing budget cuts or that the library is compensating for budget cuts with the fee. Similarly, the announcement says nothing about the library's Internet costs, so it is impossible to conclude logically that the library is attempting to offset its own Internet fees.

39. C: Raoul will need the computer for a total of 90 minutes. The first 30 minutes are free, so Raoul will need to be prepared to pay for 60 minutes. This is equal to four intervals of 15 minutes. Each 15-minute interval costs $3, so Raoul will need to pay $12 for his Internet usage at the library.

40. D: Good Karma Salon & Spa specifically notes that it offers haircuts, coloring, and nail services. Based on the information in the telephone book, then, this will likely be the best choice for Genevieve. The Sérénité Spa advertisement states that the business offers "all spa services," but does not specify what those services are in the same way that the Good Karma Salon & Spa advertisement does. Angel Cuts and Perfect Endings appear in the hair salon section. Therefore, while they likely offer haircuts and coloring, they may not offer nail services. Furthermore, there is nothing in these ads to suggest that manicures and pedicures are offered at these locations.

41. C: Natural Nails advertises that it uses no harsh chemicals or toxic products, so this is Genevieve's best option to avoid another allergic reaction. Nails by Manhattan and Hands to Envy make no comment about the chemical content of their products, so Genevieve should probably avoid these places. Perfect Endings is a hair salon, not a nail salon.

42. A: Hair and a Spare is located at 274 Finch, while Natural Nails is located at 285 Finch. These businesses would almost certainly be in the same shopping center, if not right next door to each other. Perfect Endings and Hands to Envy are located on the same street, but the address numbers are so far apart that these two businesses are likely not in the same shopping center. The same is true for Nails by Manhattan and Airbrushed Tans. Angel Cuts and Cannes Tan are located on different streets.

43. C: Although it never specifically addresses the babysitter, the directions are clearly instructions for how to take care of a little girl. A mother or father would not need this information written down in such detail, but a babysitter might. You can infer the answer in this case.

44. D: You cannot assume gender, and the note never indicates whether the writer is male or female. You can tell that the writer is the main caretaker of the child in question, so "parent" is the best choice in this case. A teacher or nurse might be able to write such a note, but parent is probably more likely, making it the best choice.

45. B: The information in the passage lets you know that only the serving team can score. This rule is different in different leagues, so it is important to read the passage instead of going by what you know from your own life.

46. D: Although any number of people could play in a volleyball game, the passage mentions that the entire class could participate in a game. Do all of them have to participate? No. But that wasn't the question.

47. A: The referee might yell any number of things, but only "side out" is mentioned in the passage.

48. C: In volleyball, all that is needed in terms of equipment is a ball and a net. Answer choice E, 15 points, is the number of points needed to win.

Mathematics Answer Explanations

1. C: According to the problem statement, 60% of the class wanted to work with the elderly. Therefore, convert 60% to a fraction by using the following steps:

$$60\% = \frac{60}{100}$$

Now simplify the above fraction using a greatest common factor of 20.

$$\frac{60}{100} = \frac{3}{5}$$

2. B: Since 35% of the staff will take vacation days, only 100% − 35% = 65% of the staff is available to work. Of the remaining 65%, only 20% are certified to work in the neonatal unit. Therefore multiply 65% by 20% using these steps:
Convert 65% and 20% into decimals by dividing both numbers by 100.

$$\frac{65}{100} = 0.65 \text{ and } \frac{20}{100} = 0.20$$

Now multiply 0.65 by 0.20 to get
$$(0.65)(0.20) = 0.13$$
Now convert 0.13 to a percentage by multiplying by 100.
$$(0.13)(100) = 13\%$$

3. B: The patient's dosage must decrease by 30%. So calculate 30% of 340:
$$(0.30)(340 \text{ mg}) = 102 \text{ mg}$$
Now subtract the 30% decrease from the original dosage.
$$340 \text{ mg} - 102 \text{ mg} = 238 \text{ mg}$$

4. C: Since 70% of the patients in the study were women, 30% of the patients were men. Calculate the number of male patients by multiplying 100 by 0.30.
$$(100)(0.30) = 30$$
Of the 30 male patients in the study, 10% were overweight as children. So 90% were not overweight. Multiply 30 by 0.90 to get the final answer.
$$(30)(0.90) = 27$$

5. C: If the incoming class has 100 students, then $\frac{3}{4}$ of those students will major in nursing.
$$(100)\left(\frac{3}{4}\right) = 75$$
So 75 students will major in nursing but only $\frac{1}{5}$ of that 75 will complete the nursing program.
$$(75)\left(\frac{1}{5}\right) = 15$$
Therefore, 15 students will complete the program.

6. A: The first midwife receives $2000 per month, and she uses $\frac{2}{5}$ of that amount for rent and utilities.
$$(\$2000)\left(\frac{2}{5}\right) = \$800) = \$$$
So the midwife pays $800 for rent and utilities, which leaves her with
$$\$2000 - \$800 = \$1200$$
The midwife divides the remaining $1200 in half.
$$\frac{\$1200}{2} = \$600$$
The midwife saves $600 and buys medical supplies with the remaining $600.

7. A: The second midwife budgets $\frac{1}{2}$ of her loan for an office administrator plus another $\frac{1}{10}$ of her loan for office supplies. So add $\frac{1}{2}$ and $\frac{1}{10}$ by first finding a common denominator.
$$\frac{1}{2} = \frac{5}{10}$$
$$\frac{5}{10} + \frac{1}{10} = \frac{6}{10}$$
Now simplify $\frac{6}{10}$ by using the greatest common factor of 6 and 10, which is 2.
$$6 \div 2 = 3 \text{ and } 10 \div 2 = 5$$
Therefore, $\frac{6}{10} = \frac{3}{5}$.

8. D: First add all expenses for the third midwife. Then subtract her total expenses from $2000.
$$\$900 + \$200 + \$100 = \$1200$$
$$\$2000 - \$1200 = \$800$$

9. C: The ratio of her savings to the rent is 1:2, which means that for every $2 she pays in rent, she saves $1 for the purchase of an office building. To calculate the amount the fourth midwife saves for the purchase of a building, divide $800 by 2.

$$\frac{\$800}{2} = \$400$$

10. C: Each midwife contributed about $500 towards the ultrasound purchase.

$$\$500 + \$500 + \$500 + \$500 = \$2000$$

11. B: To obtain the new dosage, subtract 80 mg from the original dosage of 310 mg.

$$310 \text{ mg} - 80 \text{ mg} = 230 \text{ mg}$$

12. C: Find $\frac{1}{7}$ of 100 by multiplying

$$(100)\left(\frac{1}{7}\right) = \frac{100}{7} = 14.2857$$

$\frac{100}{7}$ is an improper fraction. Convert the fraction to a decimal and round to the nearest hundredth to get 14.29.

13. A: The Roman numeral system requires adding or subtracting the individual digits in order to obtain the full number. The X equals 10. So XX means add 10 + 10 to get 20. The I equals 1 and V equals 5. However, since the I is placed directly before the V, subtract 5 – 1 to get 4. Finally, add 20 + 4 to get 24.

14. C: Susan receives $40,000. First she contributes 10% of her salary to a retirement account.

$$(\$40,000)(0.10) = \$4,000$$
$$\$40,000 - \$4,000 = \$36,000$$

After contributing to her retirement account, Susan has $36,000 left. Then she pays 25% in taxes.

$$(\$36,000)(0.25) = \$9,000$$
$$\$36,000 - \$9,000 = \$27,000$$

After paying taxes, Susan has $27,000 left. Finally, she pays $30 each month for health insurance. Calculate the annual amount Susan pays for health insurance, and subtract this amount from her remaining salary.

$$(\$30)(12) = \$360$$
$$\$27,000 - \$360 = \$26,640$$

15. D: To determine the total cost of Susan's outfit, add all her purchases.

$$\$69.99 + \$39.99 + \$34.76 = \$144.65$$

16. B: The beginning balance for the account was $300.00. Then two purchases were made. So subtract those purchase amounts from the beginning balance.

$$\$300.00 - \$3.56 - \$132.61 = \$163.83$$

Next, a deposit was made into the account. So add the amount of the deposit to get the ending balance.

$$\$163.83 + \$75.33 = \$239.16$$

17. A: Apply the order of operations to solve this problem. Multiplication and division are computed first from left to right. Then addition and subtraction are computed next from left to right.

$$2 + (2)(2) - 2 \div 2 =$$
$$2 + 4 - 2 \div 2 =$$
$$2 + 4 - 1 =$$
$$6 - 1 =$$
$$5$$

18. C: The office manager will order 2 cupcakes for each person and 50 people will attend the event.

$$(2)(50) = 100$$

Therefore, the manager will order 100 cupcakes. Each cupcake costs \$1.75. Calculate the total cost for cupcakes.

$$(100)(\$1.75) = \$175.00$$

19. B: Compare and order the rational numbers by finding a common denominator for all three fractions. The least common denominator for 3, 5, and 15 is 15. Now convert the fractions with different denominators into fractions with a common denominator.

$$\frac{4}{15} = \frac{4}{15}$$
$$\frac{2}{5} = \frac{6}{15}$$
$$\frac{1}{3} = \frac{5}{15}$$

Now that all three fractions have the same denominator, order them from smallest to largest by comparing the numerators.

$$\frac{4}{15} < \frac{5}{15} < \frac{6}{15}$$

Since $\frac{4}{15}$ of the patients are in Group Alpha, this group has the smallest number of patients. The next largest group has $\frac{5}{15}$ of the patients, which is Group Gamma. The largest group has $\frac{6}{15}$ of the patients, which is Group Beta.

20. A: Solve the equation for x.

$$2x + 6 = 14$$
$$2x = 14 - 6$$
$$2x = 8$$
$$x = \frac{8}{2}$$
$$x = 4$$

21. D: Add the polynomials by combining all the like terms, which have the same variable. In other words, combine all the x terms and then combine all the y terms.

$$4x + 2x + 4x + 2x = 12x$$
$$8y + 6y + 2y + 4y = 20y$$

Since $12x$ and $20y$ are different terms, the final answer is

$$12x + 20y$$

22. A: During week 1, Nurse Cameron worked 5 shifts.
$$\text{shifts for week } 1 = 5$$
During week 2, she worked twice as many shifts as she did during week 1.
$$\text{shifts for week } 2 = (2)(5)$$
During week 3, she added 4 shifts to the number of shifts she worked during week 2.
$$\text{shifts for week } 3 = (2)(5) + 4$$

23. C: Use the order of operations to solve this problem. Also remember that the absolute value of a number is always positive.
$$|(3)(-4)| + (3)(4) - 1 =$$
$$|-12| + (3)(4) - 1 =$$
$$12 + 12 - 1 =$$
$$24 - 1 =$$
$$23$$

24. B: The graph presented in choice B has the correct data and correct axes. Choice A has incorrect data. For example, physicians do not work 40 hours per week. Choice C has incorrect labels for the axes. The label, "Average hours worked per week," refers to numbers, and the label, "Hospital Staff," refers to people. Choice C has incorrect data and incorrect axes labels.

25. The correct answer is a. The section marked "Residents" takes up the largest amount of the circle graph. Therefore, the residents work the most amount of time.

26. D: The variables are the objects the graph measures. In this case, the graph measures the Hospital Staff and the Average hours worked per week. The dependent variable changes with the independent variable. Here, the average hours worked per week depends on the particular type of hospital staff. Therefore, the dependent variable is Average hours worked per week and the dependent variable is Hospital Staff.

27. D: The prefix, milli-, means 1000th. In this case,
$$1 \text{ g} = 1000 \text{ mg}$$
Therefore,
$$(5)(1 \text{ g}) = (5)(1000 \text{ mg})$$
$$5 \text{ g} = (5)(1000 \text{ mg})$$
$$5 \text{ g} = 5000 \text{ mg}$$

28. C: A small apple weighs about 100 g. Choice A, 1 mg, is much too small, and 0.001 g is the same as 1 mg. Choice D, 1000 kg, is much too large.

29. C: The meter is the only unit in the list used to describe length. The gram and pound are used to measure mass and weight, respectively, and the liter describes volume.

30. B: Each segment between marks in the figure is 2 cm long, and 3 segments are between 1 and 4. Therefore the total distance between 1 and 4 is
$$(2 \text{ cm})(3) = 6 \text{ cm}$$

31. D: Integers include all positive and negative whole numbers and the number zero. The product of three integers must be an integer, so you can eliminate any answer choice that is not a whole number: choices (A) and (C). The product of two even integers is even. The product of even and odd integers is even. The only even choice is 24.

32. C: Divide the mg the child should receive by the number of mg in 0.8 ml to determine how many 0.8 ml doses the child should receive: $\frac{240}{80} = 3$. Multiply the number of doses by 0.8 to determine how many ml the child should receive: $3 \times 0.8 = 2.4$ ml

33. B: The chart indicates that each x value must be tripled to equal the corresponding y value, so $y = 3x$. One way you can determine this is by plugging corresponding pairs of x and y into the answer choices.

34. D: Use the following proportion: $\dfrac{1 \text{ in}}{45 \text{ miles}} = \dfrac{3.2 \text{ in}}{x \text{ miles}}$

Cross multiply: $x = (45)(3.2) = 144$

Science Answer Explanations

1. C: The circulatory system circulates materials throughout the entire body. The heart is part of this system, since it is responsible for pumping blood that carries these materials. The kidneys are part of the urinary system. The lungs belong to the respiratory system, and the stomach is part of the digestive system.

2. B: The digestive system helps the body process food. The stomach, mouth, and esophagus all participate in food digestion. The brain, however, is part of the nervous system.

3. A: The nervous system is the body's communication center. The body uses the respiratory system to breathe, and blood is transported by the circulatory system. The digestive system breaks down food for the body.

4. D: The respiratory system uses the lungs, diaphragm, trachea, and bronchi to help the body breathe. The nervous system is the body's center of communication. The circulatory system transports materials through the body, and the digestive system processes food.

5. A: The immune system helps protect the body from bacteria, viruses, infections, and other elements that could cause illness. The digestive and nervous systems are discussed in the explanations for questions 3 and 4. The urinary system helps the body expel liquid waste.

6. A: The human body has five types of bones: long bones, short bones, irregular bones, flat bones, and sesamoid bones. While bones may be dense, this is not a major category of bones in the body.

7. B: Sesamoid bones are embedded in tendons. Choice D, vertical bones, is not a major bone type. Long bones contain a long shaft, and flat bones are thin and curved.

8. C: An increase in the birth rate would lead to growth in the population. Fatal disease, migration to Europe, and increased death rate would cause the population to decline.

9. D: Among other factors, fertility in women is adversely affected by smoking, stress, and alcohol consumption. Therefore, women who desire optimum fertility should consume alcohol in moderation, refrain from smoking, and avoid stressful situations.

10. B: If scientists created a cure for cancer, people who otherwise would have died from cancer would continue to live. Therefore, the population would most likely increase.

11. A: Each year, 3% of the population in country Q leaves but only 1% returns. Therefore, more people leave each year than move back, and the population steadily declines.

12. A: The process of natural selection describes how animals survive by adapting to their environment. The animals that survive produce offspring who have the same survival skills. In this case, the giraffes with long necks were able to survive by eating a food source that may not have been available to animals that usually ate food near the ground. The giraffes with long necks then produced offspring with long necks who could eat from this higher food source.

13. D: The term "*Homo sapiens*" is used by scientists to classify humans. In the biological classification system, *Homo* is the genus and *sapiens* designates the species.

14. C: Mitochondria are often called the power house of the cell because they provide energy for the cell to function. The nucleus is the control center for the cell. The cell membrane surrounds the cell and separates the cell from its environment. Cytoplasm is the thick fluid within the cell membrane that surrounds the nucleus and contains organelles.

15. B: Ribosomes are organelles that help synthesize proteins within the cell. Cilia and flagella are responsible for cell movement. The cell membrane helps the cell maintain its shape and protects it from the environment. Lysosomes have digestive enzymes.

16. B: Cells differentiate so that simple, less specialized cells can become highly specialized cells. For example, humans are multicellular organisms who undergo cell differentiation numerous times. Cells begin as simple zygotes after fertilization and then differentiate to form a myriad of complex tissues and systems before birth.

17. C: Both meiosis and mitosis occur in humans, other animals, and plants. Mitosis produces cells that are genetically identical, and meiosis produces cells that are genetically different. Only mitosis occurs asexually.

18. B: Photosynthesis describes the process plants use to generate food from sunlight, carbon dioxide, and water. It does not occur in animals. Respiration is the process by which oxygen is used to release energy from glucose, producing carbon dioxide. It occurs in both plants and animals, though in plants the amount of oxygen produced by photosynthesis is generally more than that used by respiration.

19. B: DNA is the primary carrier of genetic information in most cells. RNA serves as a messenger that transmits genetic information from DNA to the cytoplasm of the cell.

20. B: Genetic mutations are changes in DNA that occur spontaneously at low rates. Genetic mutations rarely occur at fast rates. If the DNA remains the same, no mutation occurs.

21. C: After cell division, the daughter cells should be exact copies of the parent cells. Therefore, the DNA should replicate, or make an exact copy of itself, so that each daughter cell will have the full amount of DNA.

22. A: Genes are the molecular units that enable parents to pass hereditary traits on to their offspring. The blood, organs, and hair all contain the genes that makeup the offspring, but these are not basic molecular units.

23. A: Both DNA and RNA are made up of 4 nucleotide bases. Both DNA and RNA contain cytosine, guanine, and adenine. However, DNA contains thymine and RNA contains uracil. Choice B is incorrect because DNA and RNA do not have the same 4 nucleotides, and choices C and D are incorrect because neither DNA nor RNA contains 6 nucleotides. Furthermore, DNA has a double helix structure, and RNA has a single helix structure.

24. B: The genotype describes a person's genetic makeup. The phenotype describes a person's observable characteristics. Among the choices, the CFTR gene refers to genetic makeup while the other choices all describe traits that are observable.

25. D: The complete Punnett square is shown below.

	B	b
B	BB	Bb
b	Bb	bb

Because male pattern baldness is a recessive gene, the offspring would need the *bb* gene combination in order to inherit this trait. Possibility 4 corresponds to the *bb* gene combination.

26. D: Refer to the complete Punnett square in the explanation for question 25. Because male pattern baldness is recessive, the offspring would need the *bb* gene combination in order to inherit this trait. Therefore, any offspring with the *B* gene will have a full head of hair. Possibilities 1, 2, and 3 all have the *B* gene.

27. C: The sun is the celestial body that serves as a major external source of heat, light, and energy for Earth. Mars is a planet and the Big Dipper is a constellation. The moon only reflects the light of the sun and is not an energy source for Earth.

28. A: Oxidation is half of a redox (oxidation-reduction) reaction. Oxidation refers to losing electrons and reduction refers to gaining electrons. The two reactions always occur in pairs. In this case, an example of an oxidation reaction is copper losing 2 electrons.

29. A: A catalyst increases the rate of a chemical reaction without becoming part of the net reaction. Therefore, chemical C increases the rate of the reaction between A and B. The catalyst does not change the chemicals within the reaction.

30. B: Enzymes are protein molecules produced by living organisms. Enzymes serve as catalysts for certain biological reactions.

31. C: The pH of acids is less than 7, and the pH of bases is greater than 7. A substance with a pH equal to 7 is neutral.

32. A: An ionic bond occurs between atoms when one atom donates valence electrons to another atom that receives those electrons. In this case, sodium donates an electron to chlorine, forming an ionic bond between the two atoms.

33. D: Water molecules contain hydrogen and oxygen atoms that are covalently bonded. Water molecules do not have ionic bonds. Also, water has a neutral pH of 7.

34. B: In general, the faster an object is moving, the more kinetic energy it possesses. In choices A, C, and D, the ball is not moving, so it has no kinetic energy. In choice B, the ball is in motion, so it does have some kinetic energy in this case.

35. C: The atom is negatively charged. Neutrons have no charge. Protons have positive charge and electrons have negative charge equal in magnitude to the positive charge of the proton. Because the atom has more electrons than protons, the atom has a negative charge.

36. D: The nucleus contains protons and neutrons while electrons orbit the nucleus of the atom. Positrons are not a major component of an atom, and "negatron" is just an obsolete term for an electron.

37. A: A covalent bond is formed between atoms that share electrons. For example, the hydrogen and oxygen atoms in water have covalent bonds because they share their valence electrons.

38. D: The atomic number equals the number of protons and the number of electrons in an atom. Since Be has an atomic number of 4, it has 4 protons and 4 electrons. H has the fewest protons and electrons, as denoted by its atomic number of 1.

39. B: Liquids are free flowing and take on the shape of their container. Solids are rigid and fixed. Therefore, the atoms in a solid have a fixed structure.

40. C: Vaporization is the process of changing from a liquid to a gas. For instance, water vaporizes when boiled to create steam. Freezing is the process of changing from a liquid to a solid. Condensation describes changing from a gas to a liquid, and sublimation is the process of changing from a solid to a gas.

41. C: The nurse wants to investigate her patients' body temperatures. A thermometer is the only tool in the list that will help measure the temperature of a person's body.

42. A: The researcher should use statistical analysis to understand trends in the data. Different statistics tools can help manage and examine large data sets. The researcher would probably miss important correlations by looking at the individual data points, and eliminating most of the data would defeat the purpose of conducting the study. Simply staring at the data would not be helpful.

43. B: Based on the evidence, the most likely explanation for fly larvae in the spoiled food is that flies laid their eggs in the food. When the food was left out in the open, the flies had access to it and laid their eggs. However, when the food was in a sealed container, the flies could not lay their eggs in the food. Hence, the spoiled food in the sealed container had no fly larvae.

44. D: Longer life expectancy could be explained by any or all of the alternatives presented. Advances in medical technology, basic cleanliness, and vaccines could all help people live longer in the 21st century.

45. C: A scientific argument should be based on measurable and observable facts such as the patient's current symptoms and health history. Discussing the patient's appearance or the doctor's feelings does not communicate a scientific argument. While insurance may be a factor in most healthcare systems, the status of the patient's insurance does not communicate a scientific argument that justifies the need for the test.

46. B: The best reason to conduct this investigation is so the board can determine if the ER is understaffed. Although the board may want to feel good, this is not a good reason to conduct an investigation. While advertising may be important to the success of the hospital, having the proper staff in the emergency is more critical than advertising.

47. A: Technology should be used in scientific research for several reasons. Among the items in this list, the best reason is the large amount of data that technology allows researchers to collect and analyze. While technology does allow researchers to create nice pictures and spend more time with their families, these reasons are secondary to data collection and analysis.

48. A: Although some unscrupulous researchers may use mathematics to sway research outcomes, this is not a reason to include math in scientific research. Creating measurable research goals, seeking objective data analysis, and discovering trends and patterns are all good reasons to include mathematics in scientific research.

49. D: Of the given structures, veins have the lowest blood pressure. *Veins* carry oxygen-poor blood from the outlying parts of the body to the heart. An *artery* carries oxygen-rich blood from the heart to the peripheral parts of the body. An *arteriole* extends from an artery to a capillary. A *venule* is a tiny vein that extends from a capillary to a larger vein.

50. C: Of the four heart chambers, the left ventricle is the most muscular. When it contracts, it pushes blood out to the organs and extremities of the body. The right ventricle pushes blood into the lungs. The atria, on the other hand, receive blood from the outlying parts of the body and transport it into the ventricles. The basic process works as follows: Oxygen-poor blood fills the right atrium and is pumped into the right ventricle, from which it is pumped into the pulmonary artery and on to the lungs. In the lungs, this blood is oxygenated. The blood then reenters the heart at the left atrium, which when full pumps into the left ventricle. When the left ventricle is full, blood is pushed into the aorta and on to the organs and extremities of the body.

51. A: The *cerebrum* is the part of the brain that interprets sensory information. It is the largest part of the brain. The cerebrum is divided into two hemispheres, connected by a thin band of tissue called the corpus callosum. The *cerebellum* is positioned at the back of the head, between the brain stem and the cerebrum. It controls both voluntary and involuntary movements. The *medulla oblongata* forms the base of the brain. This part of the brain is responsible for blood flow and breathing, among other things.

52. C: *Collagen* is the protein produced by cartilage. Bone, tendon, and cartilage are all mainly composed of collagen. *Actin* and *myosin* are the proteins responsible for muscle contractions. Actin makes up the thinner fibers in muscle tissue, while myosin makes up the thicker fibers. Myosin is the most numerous cell protein in human muscle. *Estrogen* is one of the steroid hormones produced mainly by the ovaries. Estrogen motivates the menstrual cycle and the development of female sex characteristics.

53. C: The parasympathetic nervous system is responsible for lowering the heart rate. It slows down the heart rate, dilates the blood vessels, and increases the secretions of the digestive system. The central nervous system is composed of the brain and the spinal cord. The sympathetic nervous system is a part of the autonomic nervous system; its role is to oppose the actions taken by the parasympathetic nervous system. So, the sympathetic nervous system accelerates the heart, contracts the blood vessels, and decreases the secretions of the digestive system.

54. A: An adult inhales 500 mL of air in an average breath. Interestingly, humans can inhale about eight times as much air in a single breath as they do in an average breath. People tend to take a larger breath after making a larger inhalation. This is one reason that many breathing therapies, for instance those incorporated into yoga practice, focus on making a complete exhalation. The process of respiration is managed by the autonomic nervous system. The body requires a constant replenishing of oxygen, so even brief interruptions in respiration can be damaging or fatal.

English and Language Usage Answer Explanations

1. A: Semicolons are used to separate items in a series when those items contain internal commas, such as in a listing of cities and states. Answer choice A correctly demonstrates this. Answer choice B places the semicolon between the city and its state, instead of between *each* listing of the city and its state, and this is incorrect. A comma is always used to separate a single instance of a city and a state. Answer choice C separate the items in the series with commas, but this creates confusion for the reader, since there are already commas between each city and its state. Answer choice D places commas between each item in the series, but fails to include the necessary comma between each city and its state.

2. C: The word *conscientious* tends to fall into the "frequently misspelled category," and answer choice C demonstrates the correct spelling of the word. The other answer choices fail to spell the word accurately.

3. B: Answer choice B presents the correct order of words for the sentence: They're [They are] going on vacation to their [possessive pronoun] house on Lake Chelan, and they plan to water ski and parasail while there [adverb indicating location]. The other answer choices place these words in incorrect order.

4. C: When a plural word is made possessive, the standard rule is to place the apostrophe after the final *s*, as in *jurors'*. Answer choice C correctly demonstrates this. Answer choices A and D place the possessive apostrophe within *meals* (*meal's* and *meals'*), and these forms of the word do not make sense within the context of the sentence. Answer choice B places the possessive apostrophe before the final *s*, as in *juror's*, which indicates only a single juror. This form is incorrect in the context of the sentence.

5. B: A complex sentence contains a single independent clause in addition to a dependent clause. Answer choice B opens with the dependent clause *Before Ernestine purchases a book* and ends with the independent clause *she always checks to see if the library has it*. Answer choice A is a simple sentence, as it has no dependent clause. Answer choice C is a compound sentence, because it has two independent clauses. Answer choice D is also a simple sentence, although it has a compound subject.

6. D: In the context of the sentence, it appears that Finlay's parents are attempting to *coax* him by promising a trip to his favorite toy store. Answer choice A makes little sense, as the sentence indicates Finlay's parents want him to participate in the recital. Answer choice B might work, but the promise of a trip to the toy store seems more like a reward than a punishment. Answer choice C makes no sense when added to the sentence in place of the word *cajole*.

7. C: The correct plural form of *tempo* is *tempi*. This word has an Italian root, and thus follows the pattern of other, similar words that end in *-i* in their plural form. Note also that *tempo*, meaning time, is simply the Italian form of the Latin *tempus*. (Recall the Latin expression *tempus fugit*, or "time flies.") Other Latin-based nouns ending in *-us* also take the *-i* ending when made plural: *octopus > octopi, syllabus > syllabi*, etc.

8. A: In answer choice A, *Aunt Jo* is correctly capitalized, because *aunt* identifies a specific person. The word *uncle* is not capitalized in this sentence, because the uncle's name is not added. Answer choice B fails to capitalize *Brother Mark*, as the expression clearly identifies a monk. Answer choice C fails to capitalize *Cousin Martha*. *Cousin* should be capitalized, because the word identifies a specific individual. Answer choice D fails to capitalize *Outer Banks*, which is the proper noun for a region; answer choice D also incorrectly capitalizes *Fall*. Seasons are not capitalized.

9. D: The correct pronoun for the antecedent *person* is *his or her*. The plural *their* in answer choice A is incorrect, because the word *person* is singular. Answer choice B cannot be correct, because a person is not identified as *it* in the English language. The article *the*, answer choice C, makes little sense in the context of the sentence.

10. B: Answer choice B demonstrates a comma splice, which is the use of a comma to join two independent clauses. Note that *however* is not a conjunction, and cannot join two sentences like other coordinating conjunctions (e.g., *and*, *but*, *or*, etc.) can. Answer choice A correctly uses a semicolon between the independent clauses. Answer choice C correctly uses a period between the independent clauses. Answer choice D correctly uses a comma and the coordinating conjunction *but* to join the independent clauses.

11. B: Answer choice B combines the sentences in the best way. The sentences are combined into a single sentence, and all of the details are still included. Answer choices A and D do a good job of combining the sentences, but still consist of more than one sentence. Answer choice C combines the sentences, but leaves out the part about how she "tried to find a way to attend both." There is no clear reason to leave this out, so answer choice C is not the best choice.

12. A: The correct plural form of *human* is *humans*. Despite the fact that it contains the form *man*, the plural form is not *humen*, as indicated in answer choice B. Answer choices C and D both contain apostrophes, which are not necessary in standard plural forms.

13. D: If the root *meare* means "to pass," and the word *permeate* means "to penetrate or pervade," the most likely meaning of the prefix *per-* is "through." This would yield a literal word meaning of "to pass through," which is similar in meaning to the original: "to penetrate or pervade." The phrase "to pass across" does not match the original Latin origins. Similarly, "to pass by" and "to pass with" are not consistent with the meaning of "passing through."

14. B: Anthropology is the study of human culture. Cosmetology is the study of cosmetic techniques. Etymology is the study of word meanings. Genealogy is the study of family history. All of these words would indicate that the suffix *-logy* refers to the study of something. It cannot refer to a record, since that indicates something in the past, and the words in question describe activities that are ongoing An affinity for something is not the same as a committed study of it, and each item in the question represents its own dedicated field. The suffix for "fear" is *-phobia*.

15. D: An adverb modifies a verb, and in the sentence, the word *well* modifies the verb *did* by indicating *how* Jacob did with his speech. The word *worried* is a verb. The word *about* is a preposition. The word *but* is a conjunction.

16. B: The correct version of the sentence is as follows: "Most doctors agree that there are a lot of reasons to add a daily multivitamin to the diet." Both blanks need plural verbs, the verb *agree* to modify the plural *doctors*, and the verb *are* to modify the plural *a lot*. All other answer choices include at least one singular verb, and these are therefore incorrect in the context of the sentence.

17. C: It is correct to pair a plural verb with a collective noun when that noun indicates a plural context. In answer choice C, it is clear that the faculty members are acting individually in their disagreement, so the plural verb makes sense. In answer choice A, the pronoun *neither* is singular, so the verb that accompanies it should also be singular. In answer choice B, the pronoun *all* is plural, so the accompanying verb should be plural. Similarly, in answer choice D, the pronoun *both* is plural, so the verb that accompanies it should also be plural.

18. D: The sentence suggests that the scholar was very *knowledgeable* about his subject matter; it is just that his presentation went over the students' heads. The word *authentic* suggests an external guarantee of correctness, which makes little sense in the context of the sentence. The word *arrogant* might be accurate, except that there is nothing in the sentence to suggest the guest speaker deliberately spoke over the students' heads. It is simply that his knowledge was not presented effectively given the audience. Finally, there is nothing in the sentence to suggest that the guest speaker was *faulty* in any way. Rather, he knew so much that he failed to connect with an audience that was less knowledgeable.

19. C: The word *sacrilegious* indicates a violation of sacred expectations, and wearing white to a funeral would be something that would violate the sacred expectations of many. The other answer choices are spelled incorrectly, particularly *sacreligious*, which spells the word with the correct spelling of *religious*. This is not correct, as the spelling is adjusted when joined to the other root.

20. C: Of the answer choices, the only prefix that requires hyphenation is *self-*. The other answer choices are words containing prefixes that do not require hyphens.

21. B: Answer choice B includes all of the necessary information while still removing the nominalization. All of the other answer choices include nominalization in the form of extended phrases that make the statement longer and more confusing than necessary. Additionally, answer choice D claims that the city council let residents make the decision; the original sentence claims only that the city council asked for comments from residents. Therefore, answer choice D adds inaccurate information.

22. D: Answer choice D has a plural subject, but is still a simple sentence. Answer choice A is a compound sentence, as it is composed of two independent clauses. Answer choice B consists of two independent sentences that are joined by a semicolon. (The punctuation is correct, and creates two simple sentences, not one.) Answer choice C contains a dependent clause, so it is a complex sentence.

23. D: Answer choice D is a pronoun: the subjective case *I*. Answer choice A is a helping verb. Answer choice B is an adjective. Answer choice C is an adverb.

24. A: A book title should be italicized, but the chapter titles (if the chapters *are* titled) should be placed in double quotation marks. (Double quotation marks are correct for all standard quotations in American English.) Answer choice A correctly demonstrates this. All of the other answer choices incorrectly place the book title in quotation marks, or place the chapter title in single quotation marks.

25. B: Answer choice B is the clearest and the most concise. Answer choices A and C include more than one independent clause. As the statement can function as a single independent clause, this is unnecessary. Answer choice D works, but it is not the best option in terms of style, clarity, and concision. The coordinating conjunction with the added independent clause makes the sentence more unwieldy than answer choice B.

26. B: The context of the sentence suggests that Mrs. Vanderbroek would not be delighted about any changes to her routine. Thus, answer choice B makes the most sense. Answer choice A has promise, but it does not exactly fit the meaning of the sentence. It is not that Mrs. Vanderbroek would be incapable of accepting change, but rather that she would not welcome it. Answer choices C and D indicate Mrs. Vanderbroek's overall response to changes, but they do not work as synonyms for the word *amenable*.

27. D: The words *quick, available,* and *little* are all adjectives in the sentence. *Quick* modifies *review*; *available* modifies *housing options*; *little* modifies *choice*. The word *rent* is part of the infinitive (i.e. verbal) phrase *to rent*.

28. B: Based on the context of the sentence, the word in the first blank should be in the subjective case, while the word in the second blank should be in the objective case. Only answer choice B indicates this. Answer choice A places both words in the subjective case; answer choice D places both words in the objective case. Answer choice C reverses the correct order of the words. The first is in the objective case, and the second is in the subjective case.

29. D: Answer choice D combines the six sentences into two primary sentences, and this answer choice fulfills the requirement for a combination that is "as concise as possible." Answer choice C is also two primary sentences, but they reverse the flow of thought and make the sentence less sensible. Answer choices A and B are both three primary sentences, and thus are not as concise as possible.

30. A: The form *bear* is correct in this context, because it suggests the right to carry or own arms. The form *bare* indicates an uncovered limb. The word *barre* is the French form of *bar*, and is typically used to describe a ballet barre where dancers train. The word *baire* is an alternative colloquial form that refers to a mosquito net in some parts of the United States.

31. B: The preposition *among* is not used correctly in the context of the sentence. In this case, the word *between* would be more appropriate. *Among* and *between* both mean "in the midst of some other things." However, *between* is used when there are only two other things, and *among* is used when there are more than two. For example, it would be correct to say "between first and second base" or "among several friends." In this sentence, the preposition *among* is inappropriate for describing placement amid "two treatment protocols."

32. B: To say something is sincere means that it is genuine or real. For example, saying someone showed sincere concern means that their concern was genuine, and not fake.

33. B: Describing somebody as courteous implies that they are polite and well-mannered. Polite and courteous both convey the same meaning.

34. C: If you say that you comprehend something, it is the same as saying you understand it. For example, saying you comprehend what another person is saying is the same as saying you understand them.

TEAS® Practice Test #3

Reading	Mathematics	Science	English and Language Usage
1. ___	1. ___	1. ___ 49. ___	1. ___
2. ___	2. ___	2. ___ 50. ___	2. ___
3. ___	3. ___	3. ___ 51. ___	3. ___
4. ___	4. ___	4. ___ 52. ___	4. ___
5. ___	5. ___	5. ___ 53. ___	5. ___
6. ___	6. ___	6. ___ 54. ___	6. ___
7. ___	7. ___	7. ___	7. ___
8. ___	8. ___	8. ___	8. ___
9. ___	9. ___	9. ___	9. ___
10. ___	10. ___	10. ___	10. ___
11. ___	11. ___	11. ___	11. ___
12. ___	12. ___	12. ___	12. ___
13. ___	13. ___	13. ___	13. ___
14. ___	14. ___	14. ___	14. ___
15. ___	15. ___	15. ___	15. ___
16. ___	16. ___	16. ___	16. ___
17. ___	17. ___	17. ___	17. ___
18. ___	18. ___	18. ___	18. ___
19. ___	19. ___	19. ___	19. ___
20. ___	20. ___	20. ___	20. ___
21. ___	21. ___	21. ___	21. ___
22. ___	22. ___	22. ___	22. ___
23. ___	23. ___	23. ___	23. ___
24. ___	24. ___	24. ___	24. ___
25. ___	25. ___	25. ___	25. ___
26. ___	26. ___	26. ___	26. ___
27. ___	27. ___	27. ___	27. ___
28. ___	28. ___	28. ___	28. ___
29. ___	29. ___	29. ___	29. ___
30. ___	30. ___	30. ___	30. ___
31. ___	31. ___	31. ___	31. ___
32. ___	32. ___	32. ___	32. ___
33. ___	33. ___	33. ___	33. ___
34. ___	34. ___	34. ___	34. ___
35. ___		35. ___	
36. ___		36. ___	
37. ___		37. ___	
38. ___		38. ___	
39. ___		39. ___	
40. ___		40. ___	
41. ___		41. ___	
42. ___		42. ___	
43. ___		43. ___	
44. ___		44. ___	
45. ___		45. ___	
46. ___		46. ___	
47. ___		47. ___	
48. ___		48. ___	

Section 1. Reading	Number of Questions: **48**
	Time Limit: **58 Minutes**

1. Ernestine has a short research project to complete, and her assigned topic is the history of the Globe Theatre in London. Which of the following sources would be the best starting point for Ernestine's research?
   a. Roget's Thesaurus
   b. Oxford Latin Dictionary
   c. Encyclopedia Britannica
   d. Webster's Dictionary

2. List of Romance Languages
      Latin
      French
      Spanish
      Romanian
      American
      Portuguese

Analyze the headings above. Which of the following does not belong?
   a. Spanish
   b. American
   c. French
   d. Portuguese

3. The guide words at the top of a dictionary page are *considerable* and *conspicuous*. Which of the following words is an entry on this page?
   a. consonantal
   b. consumption
   c. conserve
   d. conquistador

4. Considering the dictionary guide words above, which of the following words most likely appears on the *previous* page of the dictionary?
   a. consonantal
   b. consumption
   c. conserve
   d. conquistador

5. The heavy spring rain resulted in a <u>plethora</u> of zucchini in Kit's garden, and left her desperately giving the vegetables to anyone who was interested. Which of the following is the definition for the underlined word in the sentence?
   a. irritation
   b. quantity
   c. abundance
   d. waste

6. Follow the numbered instructions to transform the starting word into a different word.
    1. Start with the word PREVARICATE.
    2. Remove the P from the beginning of the word.
    3. Replace the first A with the final E.
    4. Remove the I from the word.
    5. Remove the C from the word.
    6. Remove the A from the word.

What is the new word?
    a. REVEST
    b. REVERT
    c. REVIEW
    d. REVERSE

---

7. Ethan works in his company's acquisitions department, and he needs to purchase 500 pens to give away to customers. He finds the following information about purchasing pens in bulk.

Company	Specialty Pens	Office in Bulk	Office Warehouse	Ballpoint & Lead
Price per unit	$.97 per pen	$45 per 50 pens	$95 per 100 pens	$1 per pen OR $99 per 100 pens

Based on the information above, which company will have the best price for 500 pens?
    a. Specialty Pens
    b. Office in Bulk
    c. Office Warehouse
    d. Ballpoint & Lead

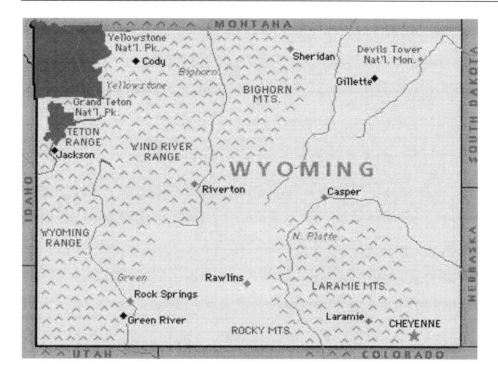

The next four questions are based on the image above.

8. On the map above, the symbol /\ indicates mountains. How many different mountain ranges are in the state of Wyoming?
   a. 3
   b. 4
   c. 5
   d. 6

9. On the map above, the star symbol indicates the state capital. Which city is the capital of Wyoming?
   a. Laramie
   b. Cheyenne
   c. Jackson
   d. Sheridan

10. On the map above, how many national parks are shown in the state of Wyoming?
   a. 2
   b. 3
   c. 4
   d. 5

11. On the map above, which states are south of Wyoming?
   a. Utah and Idaho
   b. Colorado and Utah
   c. Montana and Colorado
   d. Colorado and Nebraska

12. The warning against smoking may have been <u>tacit</u>, but Beryl instinctively knew that her mother wanted her to avoid picking up the habit. Which of the following is the definition for the underlined word in the sentence?
    a. complicated
    b. empty
    c. wordy
    d. unstated

They were known as "The Five": a group of Russian musicians who eschewed rigidly formal classical training and set out on their own to give a new artistic sound to classical music in Russia. Mily Balakirev and Cesar Cui are considered the founders of the movement, but the three who later joined them have become far more famous and respected outside, and perhaps even inside, of Russia. Modest Mussorgsky, with his passion for themes of Russian folklore and nationalism, is remembered for the piano piece *Pictures and an Exhibition*, as well as for the passionate opera *Boris Godunov*. Nikolai Rimsky-Korsakov, who spent his early years as a naval officer, had a penchant for infusing his works with the sounds of the sea. But, he might be best remembered for the hauntingly beautiful symphonic suite *Scheherazade*. Alexander Borodin balanced a career as a skilled and highly-respected chemist with his interest in classical music. He produced a number of symphonies, as well as the opera *Prince Igor*. Despite their lack of formal training and their unorthodox approach to producing classical music, The Five had an influence that reached far beyond their time. Composers such as Alexander Glazunov, Sergei Prokofiev, and Igor Stravinsky studied under Rimsky-Korsakov. Additionally, the mid-twentieth century composer Dmitri Shostakovich studied under Glazunov, creating a legacy of musical understanding that persisted well beyond the era of The Five.

The next three questions are based on the information above.

13. Which of the following describes the type of writing used in the passage?
    a. narrative
    b. persuasive
    c. expository
    d. technical

14. Which of the following is the best summary sentence for the passage?
    a. Composers such as Alexander Glazunov, Sergei Prokofiev, and Igor Stravinsky studied under Rimsky-Korsakov.
    b. Despite their lack of formal training and their unorthodox approach to producing classical music, The Five had an influence that reached far beyond their time.
    c. They were known as "The Five": a group of Russian musicians who eschewed rigidly formal classical training and set out on their own to give a new artistic sound to classical music in Russia.
    d. Mily Balakirev and Cesar Cui are considered the founders of the movement, but the three who later joined them have become far more famous and respected outside, and perhaps even inside, of Russia.

15. Based on the information in the passage, which of the composers among The Five would the author likely agree was the most influential?
    a. Alexander Glazunov
    b. Modest Mussorgsky
    c. Nikolai Rimsky-Korsakov
    d. Cesar Cui

A dictionary entry includes the following information for the word *collar*:
col‧lar [**kol**-er] *n* [Middle English, *coler*, fr. Old French *colier*, fr. Latin *collare* neckband, fr. *collum* neck]

The next three questions are based on the information above.

16. The symbol in the middle of the word *collar* indicates which of the following?
    a. emphasis
    b. spelling
    c. origin
    d. syllables

17. The bold font used in the first half of the word indicates which of the following?
    a. emphasis
    b. spelling
    c. origin
    d. syllables

18. Based on the information in the dictionary entry, what is the earliest language origin of the word *collar*?
    a. English
    b. Middle English
    c. Old French
    d. Latin

---

19. Seeing the cookie crumbs on the child's face, Ena could not believe he would tell such a barefaced lie and claim he had not eaten any cookies. Which of the following is the definition for the underlined word in the sentence?
    a. effective
    b. arrogant
    c. shameless
    d. hostile

Monarchs of England: House of Stuart
>   James I (reigned 1603-1625)
>   Charles I (reigned 1625-1649)
>   Oliver Cromwell (lord protector 1653-1658)
>   Charles II (reigned 1660-1685)
>   James II (reigned 1685-1688)
>   Mary II (reigned 1689-1694)
>   William III (reigned 1689-1702)
>   Anne (reigned 1702-1714)

The next two questions are based on the information above.

20. Analyze the headings above using the information provided in the title. Which of the following does not belong?
    a. William III
    b. Anne
    c. Charles II
    d. Oliver Cromwell

21. In the headings listed above, there are two occasions when a break occurs in the House of Stuart, and dates are missing. Before the reign of which of the following two monarchs do these breaks occur?
    a. Charles I and Charles II
    b. Charles II and Mary II
    c. Charles II and James II
    d. William III and Anne

Starting in 1856, Alfred, Lord Tennyson began publishing his compilation of Arthurian legends that became known as *Idylls of the King*. These poems were based on the earlier Medieval collection *Le Morte d'Arthur*, by Sir Thomas Malory, which dated to the middle of the 15th century. Malory's work, which is believed to be largely a translation of older French stories, was written in prose style. It combined the earlier tales into a single grouping for English readers. As the title suggests, Malory's focus was largely on the epic nature of Arthur's life. Malory discussed his birth, his rise as a prince and warrior, his quests as a knight, and his eventual death. Malory also included chapters on knights such as Lancelot and Gareth, and he discussed the relationships between Tristan and Isolde, and Lancelot and Guinevere. Instead of embracing the romance angle, however, Malory focused more on the moral elements within these stories.

Tennyson, though heavily influenced by Malory, took a different approach to the Arthurian stories. For one, he wrote them in poetry form, not prose. Additionally, Tennyson, as a Victorian poet, was more interested in the romantic qualities of the stories, and included the distinct elements of nature and elegy. *Idylls of the King* has a softer focus overall. For instance, in Malory's work, Guinevere faces execution for her adultery, and is only spared when Lancelot rides in to rescue her. In Tennyson's work, Arthur chooses to forgive Guinevere, and she chooses to spend the rest of her days doing good works in a convent. Some literary scholars believe that Tennyson was writing an allegory about social problems and the need for social justice that

existed during Tennyson's own time. Charles Dickens is remembered for doing the
same thing in his novels about the abuses of lower-class children in Victorian
England.

The next four questions are based on the information above.

22. Which of the following describes the structure of the above passage?
    a. problem-solution
    b. sequence
    c. comparison-contrast
    d. cause-effect

23. The author of the passage notes several distinctions between Tennyson and Malory. Which of
the following is not identified as a difference between the two authors?
    a. Malory wrote prose, while Tennyson wrote poetry.
    b. Malory wrote during the Medieval era, while Tennyson wrote during the Victorian era.
    c. Malory was more focused on heroism and morality, while Tennyson was more focused on
    nature and elegy.
    d. Malory wrote stories about Gareth, Tristan, and Isolde, while Tennyson focused only on
    Arthur, Lancelot, and Guinevere.

24. Which of the following sentences distracts the reader from the main focus of the passage?
    a. Malory's work, which is believed to be largely a translation of older French stories, was
    written in prose style.
    b. Instead of embracing the romance angle, however, Malory focused more on the moral
    elements within these stories.
    c. In Tennyson's work, Arthur chooses to forgive Guinevere, and she chooses to spend the rest
    of her days doing good works in a convent.
    d. Charles Dickens is remembered for doing the same thing in his novels about the abuses of
    lower-class children in Victorian England.

25. With which of the following statements would the author of the passage most likely agree?
    a. Malory and Tennyson shaped their approach to the Arthurian legends based on the defining
    qualities of their respective eras.
    b. Because *Le Morte d'Arthur* is more of a translation than a literary creation, *Idylls of the King* is
    a superior work.
    c. By undermining the moral qualities that Malory highlighted, Tennyson failed to appreciate
    the larger purpose of the stories in a Medieval context.
    d. Ultimately, Malory's influence on Tennyson was minimal, because Tennyson took a different
    approach and infused his poems with the mood of his day.

26. Regina has a severe allergy to dairy products. She is going to attend a work-related function during which lunch will be served. She requests to see the menu before the function to make sure there is something she will be able to eat. For lunch, the organizers will be serving soup, bread, and a light salad. The following soup options are available:

Egg drop soup
Lentil soup
Broccoli cheese soup
Cream of tomato soup

Which of the above options is most likely the best choice for Regina?
a. Egg drop soup
b. Lentil soup
c. Broccoli cheese soup
d. Cream of tomato soup

World War I Casualties: European Allies (1914-1918)

Country	Military Deaths	Military Wounded	Civilian Deaths (war/famine/disease)	Total Population	Percent of Population Lost
Belgium	58,637	44,686	62,000	7,400,000	1.63
France	1,397,800	4,266,000	300,000	39,600,000	4.29
Italy	651,000	953,886	589,000	35,600,000	3.48
Romania	250,000	120,000	450,000	7,500,000	9.33
Russia	2,254,369	4,950,000	1,500,000	175,100,000	2.14
United Kingdom	886,939	1,663,435	109,000	45,400,000	2.19

Sources: Commonwealth War Graves Commission, La Population de la France pendant de la guerre, United Kingdom War Office, United States War Department

The next four questions are based on the information above.

27. In terms of the percentage of its entire population, which of the following nations suffered the greatest loss during World War I?
a. France
b. Italy
c. Romania
d. Russia

28. In terms of numbers alone, which of the following nations suffered the greatest loss during World War I?
a. Belgium
b. Romania
c. Russia
d. United Kingdom

29. As a percentage of its total population, which of the following nations suffered the greatest loss of civilians during World War I?
    a. Belgium
    b. Italy
    c. Romania
    d. Russia

30. Based on the information provided about civilian deaths, which of the following most likely contributed to the largest number of civilian deaths during World War I?
    a. the sinking of the RMS *Lusitania* in 1915
    b. the trench warfare system that resulted in the "war of attrition"
    c. the development of mustard gas for the battlefield
    d. the Spanish Influenza epidemic of 1918

Announcement for all faculty members:

It has come to the university's attention that there is crowding in the faculty canteen between the hours of 11 a.m. and 1 p.m., an issue that is due to the increase in staff numbers in several faculty departments. A number of faculty members have complained that they stood in line so long that they were unable to get lunch, or did not have time to eat lunch. To offset the crowding, the university has polled the various departments about schedules, and has settled on a recommended roster for when the members of each department should visit the faculty canteen for lunch:
    Business Dept: 10.30 a.m.-11.30 a.m.
    Art Dept: 10.45 a.m.-11.45 a.m.
    Math and Science Dept: 12 p.m.-1 p.m.
    Social Sciences Dept: 12.30 p.m.-1.30 p.m.
    Humanities Dept: 1 p.m.-2 p.m.

We ask that all faculty members respect this schedule. Faculty will be expected to display a department badge before entering the canteen for lunch.

The next two questions are based on the information above.

31. Based on the information in the announcement, what might the reader assume about how the university determined the lunch schedule?
    a. The university arranged the schedule alphabetically, according to the name of each department.
    b. The university checked with the departments in advance to make sure faculty members would be amenable to the change.
    c. The university checked to see when the most faculty members from each department would be entering the canteen.
    d. The university was most concerned about crowding in the canteen, and simply decided to establish different times for each department.

32. Which best describes the final two sentences of the announcement?
    a. a friendly reminder to all faculty members to bring a badge to the canteen
    b. a word of caution to faculty members about trying to enter the canteen at the wrong time
    c. an implied suggestion that faculty members should consider getting lunch elsewhere
    d. an indication of university sanctions for faculty members who enter the canteen outside the schedule

---

During the summer, Angela read the following classics: *The Great Gatsby*, by F. Scott Fitzgerald; *Brave New World*, by Aldous Huxley; *A Passage to India*, by E.M. Forster; and "The Cask of Amontillado," by Edgar Allen Poe.

The next two questions are based on the sentence above.

33. In the statement above, several items are italicized, while only one is placed in quotation marks. According to the rules of punctuation, the following should be placed in quotation marks: article titles, book chapters, short stories, and episodes of television shows. Considering the list of works that Angela read, into which category does "The Cask of Amontillado" most likely fit?
    a. newspaper article
    b. book chapter
    c. short story
    d. television show episode

34. What is the purpose of the italics used for several of the works identified in the sentence above?
    a. to indicate a full-length published book
    b. to indicate a work of classic literature
    c. to indicate recommended summer reading
    d. to indicate books that Angela completed

35. Based on the student's <u>florid</u> complexion, Vivienne knew that his nerves were getting the better of him before the debate. Which of the following is the definition for the underlined word in the sentence?
    a. rambling
    b. flushed
    c. unclear
    d. weak

36. In a book review published in a large national newspaper, the reviewer said the book was "most likely to be enjoyed only by those with puerile fantasies." Based on this description, what can be inferred about the reviewer's opinion?
    a. The reviewer strongly recommends the book for young adults.
    b. The reviewer believes the book is inappropriate for children.
    c. The reviewer considers the book to have wide audience appeal.
    d. The reviewer feels that the book would not appeal to mature adults.

Thomas and his sister are planning to see a new science fiction film, but they have to work around their schedules. Both are free for a showing before 6 p.m. or after 10 p.m. Here are the current show times for cinemas in their area:

Twin Theatres: 6:15 p.m., 7:20 p.m., and 8:40 p.m.
Reveler Cinema: 5:45 p.m. and 7:15 p.m.
Big Screen 14: 6:00 p.m., 6:45 p.m., 9:10 p.m., and 10:05 p.m.
Best Seat in The House: 8:20 p.m., 9:55 p.m., and 11:25 p.m.

The next two questions are based on the information above.

37. Which of these cinemas does not have an option that will work for Thomas and his sister?
   a. Twin Theatres
   b. Reveler Cinema
   c. Big Screen 14
   d. Best Seat in The House

38. After an unexpected rearrangement of their schedules, Thomas and his sister realize that they will have to squeeze in the film after 10.30 p.m. Given this new information, which cinema is the best option?
   a. Twin Theatres
   b. Reveler Cinema
   c. Big Screen 14
   d. Best Seat in The House

In an effort to conserve water, the town of Audley has asked residents and businesses to water their lawns just one day a week. It has provided the following schedule based on addresses:

Monday: addresses ending in 0 and 9
Tuesday: addresses ending in 1 and 8
Wednesday: addresses ending in 2 and 7
Thursday: addresses ending in 3 and 6
Friday: addresses ending in 5
Saturday: addresses ending in 4

Businesses with suite numbers should use the final number in the suite number to determine their watering schedule.

The next three questions are based on the information above.

39. The Morgan family lives at 5487 South Elm Street. On which day of the week will they be able to water their lawn?
   a. Tuesday
   b. Wednesday
   c. Thursday
   d. Saturday

40. Everby Title Company is located at 48752 Beech Avenue, Suite 853. On which day of the week will the company be able to water its lawn?
    a. Monday
    b. Wednesday
    c. Thursday
    d. Sunday

41. The watering schedule has only one number for both Friday and Saturday. Based on the information provided, what is the most logical reason for this?
    a. There are more addresses ending with these numbers than with the other numbers.
    b. All businesses have addresses ending in these numbers, and they consume the most water.
    c. The residents at these addresses are the most likely to consume more water.
    d. The city is more concerned about water usage in the latter part of the week.

42. Sybilla is currently working three jobs in an effort to <u>aggrandize</u> herself financially and pay off her college debts. Which of the following is the definition for the underlined word in the sentence?
    a. add
    b. develop
    c. strengthen
    d. dispute

Passage 1:

    Fairy tales, fictional stories that involve magical occurrences and imaginary creatures like trolls, elves, giants, and talking animals, are found in similar forms throughout the world. This occurs when a story with an origin in a particular location spreads geographically to, over time, far-flung lands. All variations of the same story must logically come from a single source. As language, ideas, and goods travel from place to place through the movement of peoples, stories that catch human imagination travel as well through human retelling.

Passage 2:

    Fairy tales capture basic, fundamental human desires and fears. They represent the most essential form of fictionalized human experience: the bad characters are pure evil, the good characters are pure good, the romance of royalty (and of commoners becoming royalty) is celebrated, etc. Given the nature of the fairy tale genre, it is not surprising that many different cultures come up with similar versions of the same essential story.

The next four questions are based on the two passages above.

43. On what point would the authors of both passages agree?
    a. Fairy tales share a common origin.
    b. The same fairy tale may develop independently in a number of different cultures.
    c. There are often common elements in fairy tales from different cultures.
    d. Fairy tales capture basic human fears.

44. What does the "nature of the fairy tale genre" refer to in Passage 2?
    a. The representation of basic human experience
    b. Good characters being pure good and bad characters being pure evil
    c. Different cultures coming up with similar versions of the same story
    d. Commoners becoming royalty

45. Which of the following is not an example of something the author of Passage 1 claims travels from place to place through human movement?
    a. Fairy tales
    b. Language
    c. Ideas
    d. Foods

46. Which of the following is not an example of something that the author of Passage 1 states might be found in a fairy tale?
    a. Trolls
    b. Witches
    c. Talking animals
    d. Giants

What outdoorsy, family adventure can you have on a hot, summer day? How about spelunking? If you live in an area that is anywhere near a guided, lit cave, find out the hours of operation and hit the road towards it as soon as you can. Hitch up the double jogging stroller and make your way out into the wilderness, preferably with a guide, and discover the wonders of the cool, dark earth even while it is sweltering hot in the outside world. It will be 58 degrees in that cave, and you can explore inside for as long as you please. Best part? The absolutely awesome naps that the kids will take after such an exciting adventure! Be sure to bring:
- Bottled water
- Light-up tennis shoes if you have them (they look fabulous in the dark)
- Flashlights or glow sticks just for fun
- Jackets
- Changes of clothes in case of getting muddy and/or dirty

The next two questions are based on the passage above.

47. Based on the information given, what is spelunking?
    a. going in a cave
    b. an outdoor adventure
    c. walking with a double stroller
    d. a hot, summer day

48. Given the style of writing for the passage, which of the following magazines would be the best fit for this article?
    a. *Scientific Spelunking*
    b. *Family Fun Days*
    c. *Technical Caving in America*
    d. *Mud Magazine*

Section 2. Mathematics

Number of Questions: **34**

Time Limit: **51 Minutes**

1. Dr. Maya asked Nurse Andrew to recommend patients for a study about high blood pressure and high cholesterol. When Nurse Andrew analyzed his patients, he saw that $\frac{1}{10}$ of his patients had high blood pressure and normal cholesterol, $\frac{3}{5}$ had high blood pressure and high cholesterol, $\frac{1}{4}$ had normal blood pressure and high cholesterol, and $\frac{1}{20}$ had normal blood pressure and normal cholesterol. What percentage of his patients did Nurse Andrew recommend for the study?
   a. 5%
   b. 10%
   c. 25%
   d. 60%

2. Dr. Lee saw that 30% of all his patients developed an infection after taking a certain antibiotic. He further noticed that 5% of that 30% required hospitalization to recover from the infection. What percentage of Dr. Lee's patients was hospitalized after taking the antibiotic?
   a. 1.5%
   b. 5%
   c. 15%
   d. 30%

3. A patient requires a 30% increase in the dosage of her medication. Her current dosage is 270 mg. What will her dosage be after the increase?
   a. 81 mg
   b. 270 mg
   c. 300 mg
   d. 351 mg

4. A study about bulimia was conducted on 500 patients. Within that patient population 60% were women, and 20% of the men experienced some kind of childhood trauma. How many male patients in the study did NOT experience a childhood trauma?
   a. 40
   b. 100
   c. 160
   d. 200

5. University X requires some of its nursing students to take an exam before being admitted into the nursing program. In this year's class, $\frac{1}{2}$ the nursing students were required to take the exam and $\frac{3}{5}$ of those who took the exam passed the exam. If this year's class has 200 students, how many students passed the exam?
   a. 120
   b. 100
   c. 60
   d. 50

Four roommates must use their financial aid checks to pay their living expenses.
Each student receives $1000 per month.

The next five questions are based on the information above.

6. The first roommate uses $\frac{1}{4}$ of his financial aid check for the rent and utilities. Then he divides the remainder in half so that he can save $\frac{1}{2}$ the remainder. He lives off the rest. How much money does the student live off of each month?
   a. $250
   b. $375
   c. $500
   d. $1000

7. The second roommate budgets $\frac{1}{5}$ of his check for dining out plus another $\frac{1}{4}$ of his check for social activities. What is the total fraction of the second roommate's financial aid check that is spent on dining out and social activities?
   a. $\frac{1}{20}$
   b. $\frac{9}{20}$
   c. $\frac{1}{9}$
   d. $\frac{2}{9}$

8. Each month, the third roommate pays $250 for rent and utilities. Then he pays $100 for his car and insurance. Finally, he invests $25. How much money does the third roommate have left after paying these expenses?
   a. $975
   b. $750
   c. $650
   d. $625

9. The fourth roommate is saving to buy a house. So each month he puts money aside in a special house savings account. The ratio of his monthly house savings to his rent is 1:3. If he pays $270 per month in rent, how much money does he put into his house savings account each month?
   a. $90
   b. $270
   c. $730
   d. $810

10. Three of the roommates decided to combine their money to purchase a single birthday gift for their fourth roommate. The first roommate donated $12.03. The second roommate contributed $11.96, and the third roommate gave $12.06. Estimate the total amount of money the roommates used to purchase the gift.
   a. $34
   b. $35
   c. $36
   d. $37

11. A patient was exercising for 45 minutes day. However, the doctor determined that this amount of exercise was dangerous for the patient's heart. So the doctor recommended that the patient reduce his daily exercising routine by 7 minutes. How long is the patient's new daily exercising routine?
   a. 38 minutes
   b. 45 minutes
   c. 52 minutes
   d. 60 minutes

12. A lab technician took 500 milliliters of blood from a patient. The technician used $\frac{1}{6}$ of the blood for further tests. How many milliliters of blood were used for further tests? Round your answer to the nearest hundredth.
   a. 83.00
   b. 83.30
   c. 83.33
   d. 83.34

13. A patient's medical records were faxed from a hospital in the Middle East to a hospital in the USa. The patient's weight was listed in Roman numerals as LXIV kilograms. How much does the patient weigh?
   a. 34 kg
   b. 44 kg
   c. 54 kg
   d. 64 kg

14. Veronica was recently promoted to department manager for the oncology department at a local hospital. Her gross annual salary is $70,000. Veronica contributes 15% of her salary **before** taxes to a retirement account. Then she pays 30% of her remaining salary in state and federal taxes. Finally, she pays $70 per month for health insurance for her entire family. What is Veronica's annual take-home pay?
   a. $37,660
   b. $38,430
   c. $40,810
   d. $41,580

15. Veronica decided to celebrate her promotion by purchasing a new car. The base price for the car was $40,210. She paid an additional $3,015 for a surround sound system and $5,218 for a maintenance package. What was the total price of Veronica's new car?
   a. $50,210
   b. $48,443
   c. $43,225
   d. $40,210

16. Use the following table from a savings account statement to determine the ending balance in the account.

Transaction description	Amount
Beginning balance	$503.81
Deposit money with bank teller	$125.00
Withdrawal using ATM	$215.00
Monthly interest earned	$5.38
Ending balance	??

    a. $419.19
    b. $503.81
    c. $599.19
    d. $849.19

---

17. Complete the following equation:
$$2 + (2)(4) - 4 \div 2 = ?$$
    a. 3
    b. 5
    c. 6
    d. 8

---

18. The pediatric ward of a hospital is hosting a holiday party for the children and their families. For each group of 4 people who RSVP for the party, the hospital staff will order 1 medium pizza and 8 holiday cupcakes. Each medium pizza costs $9.50, and each cupcake costs $2.75. If 160 people RSVP for the event, how much money will the hospital staff spend on pizza?
    a. $380
    b. $880
    c. $950
    d. $1520

---

19. Based on their prescribing habits, a set of doctors was divided into three groups: $\frac{1}{3}$ of the doctors were placed in Group X because they always prescribed medication. $\frac{5}{12}$ of the doctors were placed in Group Y because they never prescribed medication. $\frac{1}{4}$ of the doctors were placed in Group Z because they sometimes prescribed medication. Order the groups from largest to smallest, according to the number of doctors in each group.
    a. Group X, Group Y, Group Z
    b. Group Z, Group Y, Group X
    c. Group Z, Group X, Group Y
    d. Group Y, Group X, Group Z

20. Solve the following equation:

$$\frac{2y}{10} + 5 = 25$$

    a. $y = 25$
    b. $y = 100$
    c. $y = 150$
    d. $y = 200$

---

21. Subtract polynomial #2 from polynomial #1.

    Polynomial #1: $8x + 7y + 6z$
    Polynomial #2: $3z + 4y + 5x$

    a. $5x + 3y + z$
    b. $5xz + 3y + xz$
    c. $3x + 3y + 3z$
    d. $11x + 11y + 11z$

---

22. During January, Dr. Lewis worked 20 shifts. During February, she worked three times as many shifts as she did during January. During March, she worked half the number of shifts she worked during February. Which equation below describes the number of shifts Dr. Lewis worked in March?

    a. $\text{shifts} = 20 + 3 + \frac{1}{2}$
    b. $\text{shifts} = (20)(3)\left(\frac{1}{2}\right)$
    c. $\text{shifts} = (20)(3) + \frac{1}{2}$
    d. $\text{shifts} = 20 + (3)\left(\frac{1}{2}\right)$

---

23. Solve the following expression.

$$|2 - 10| + (2)(10) - 5$$

    a. 7
    b. 15
    c. 20
    d. 23

---

24. Which circle graph accurately describes the data presented in the table below?

Nurse specialties	Number of nurses
Anesthesia	60
Midwifery	30
Pediatrics	175
Geriatrics	100

a.

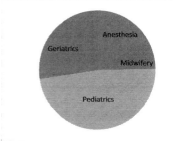

b.

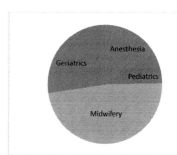

c.

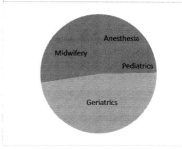

d.

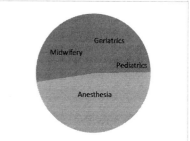

25. According to the bar graph below, which specialty has the least number of nurses?

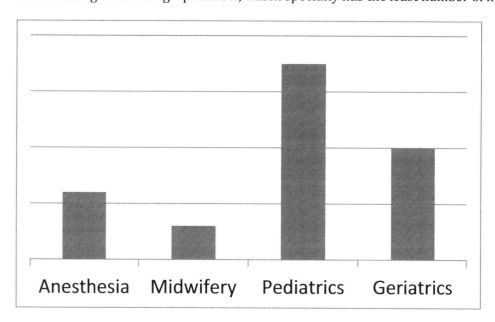

    a. Anesthesia
    b. Midwifery
    c. Pediatrics
    d. Geriatrics

26. What is the independent variable in the graph below?

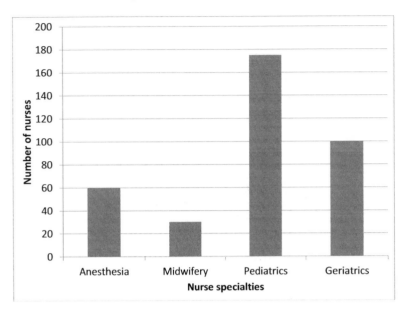

a. Anesthesia
b. Geriatrics
c. Nurse specialties
d. Number of nurses

27. How many centimeters are in 7 meters?
a. 7 m = 7 cm
b. 7 m = 70 cm
c. 7 m = 700 cm
d. 7 m = 7000 cm

28. About how long is the average human eyelash?
a. 1 nanometer
b. 1 centimeter
c. 1 meter
d. 1 kilometer

29. Which tool would most likely be used to measure the circumference of an infant's head?
a. tape measure
b. scale
c. thermometer
d. stethoscope

30. Use the figure below to determine the distance between marks 1 and 3. Each segment between marks is the same length.

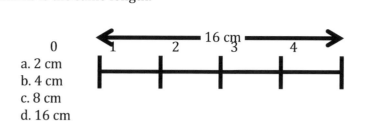

a. 2 cm
b. 4 cm
c. 8 cm
d. 16 cm

City X (250)	Profession	City Y (183)
74	Doctor	55
121	Registered Nurse	87
14	Administrator	9
15	Maintenance	11
6	Pharmacist	5
4	Radiologist	2
2	Physical Therapist	2
1	Speech Pathologist	1
13	Other	11
	Gender	
153	Male	93
97	Female	90
	Age	
24	Youngest	22
73	Oldest	77
	Ethnicity	
51	African American	42
50	Asian American	27
45	Hispanic American	35
47	Caucasian	37
57	Other	42
	Years on Staff	
64	0-5 32	
63	5-10	41
57	10-15	67
47	15-20	30
14	20-25	19
5	More than 25	5
	Number of Patient Complaints	
202	0	161
43	1-4	21
5	5-10	1
0	More than 10	0

Profile of Staff at Mercy Hospital in City X and Mercy Hospital in City Y
Total Combined Staff: 433

The next four questions are based on the previous information.

31. Which percentage is greatest?
    a. The percentage of Asian Americans to staff as a whole in City X?
    b. The percentage of staff members who have been on staff 10-15 years to staff as a whole in City X?
    c. The percentage of Doctors to staff as a whole in City X and City Y?
    d. The percentage of staff with 1-4 complaints to staff as a whole in City Y?

32. If all Caucasian staff members in City Y have been on staff between 5-10 years, how many non-Caucasian staff members in City Y have been on staff 5-10 years?
    a. 0
    b. 4
    c. 37
    d. 41

33. Approximately what percentage more staff members in City Y are female than in City X?
    a. 5
    b. 10
    c. 15
    d. 20

34. According to the chart, the percentage of staff who have received zero complaints is
    a. greater in City X than in City Y
    b. greater in City Y than in City X
    c. the same in City X and in City Y
    d. growing in both City X and City Y

Section 3. Science	Number of Questions: 54
	Time Limit: 66 Minutes

1. Which of the following items is NOT part of the circulatory system?
   a. Kidneys
   b. Heart
   c. Blood
   d. Blood vessels

2. Which of the following items belongs to the digestive system?
   a. Spine
   b. Lungs
   c. Brain
   d. Stomach

3. Which system below is the center of communication for the body?
   a. Respiratory system
   b. Nervous system
   c. Digestive system
   d. Circulatory system

4. Which item below best describes the primary function of the respiratory system?
   a. The respiratory system helps carry blood throughout the body.
   b. The respiratory system helps break down food for the body.
   c. The respiratory system helps the body breathe.
   d. The respiratory system helps send messages throughout the body.

5. Which of the following items is NOT a primary function of a healthy immune system?
   a. The immune system helps the body avoid infections.
   b. The immune system detects infections.
   c. The immune system eliminates infections.
   d. The immune system creates infections.

6. The spine and hips belong to which of the following bone types?
   a. Curvy bones
   b. Irregular bones
   c. Flat bones
   d. Long bones

7. Long bones are one of the five major types of bone in the human body. All of the following bones are long bones, EXCEPT
    a. Thighs
    b. Forearms
    c. Ankles
    d. Fingers

8. The population of the United States is directly influenced by all the following factors EXCEPT:
    a. Education
    b. Immigration
    c. Births
    d. Deaths

9. Which of the following factors would have NO influence on birth rates within a given population?
    a. The age of the women in the population
    b. The health of the women in the population
    c. The fertility of the women in the population
    d. All of these factors would influence birth rates within a given population.

10. Which of the following would most likely cause the population of the United States to increase?
    a. Women stop having children so they can focus on their careers.
    b. The government forces all adult males to join the military.
    c. Scientists discontinue all research to find cures for deadly diseases.
    d. Scientists create a cure for cancer.

11. Within a certain population, every time 1 person dies, 2 babies are born. How is this population most likely changing over time?
    a. The population is decreasing.
    b. The population is increasing.
    c. The population is remaining the same.
    d. The population has reached a steady state.

12. Which of the following scenarios does NOT describe the process of natural selection?
    a. The fastest zebras avoid being eaten by predators. Therefore, they live to produce offspring that are also fast runners.
    b. The polar bears with the thickest fur coats survive the harsh winters. Therefore, they live to produce offspring who also have thick fur coats.
    c. Animals that are born blind are soon eaten by predators. Therefore, they do not live to produce other animals that may be born blind.
    d. All of the above scenarios describe the process of natural selection.

13. Consider the categories of the biological classification system. Which choice below lists categories from broadest to most specific?
    a. Phylum, kingdom, genus, species
    b. Kingdom, phylum, genus, species
    c. Genus, kingdom, phylum, species
    d. Genus, species, phylum, kingdom

14. Which part of the cell serves as the control center for all cell activity?
    a. Nucleus
    b. Cell membrane
    c. Cytoplasm
    d. Mitochondria

15. What are the cellular functions of cilia and flagella?
    a. Cilia and flagella are responsible for cell movement.
    b. Cilia and flagella synthesize proteins.
    c. Cilia and flagella help protect the cell from its environment.
    d. Cilia and flagella have enzymes that help with digestion.

16. What is the process by which simple cells become highly specialized cells?
    a. Cellular complication
    b. Cellular specialization
    c. Cellular differentiation
    d. Cellular modification

17. How does meiosis differ from mitosis?
    a. Meiosis is used to repair the body. Mitosis is used to break down the body.
    b. Meiosis is used for asexual reproduction of single-celled organisms. Mitosis is used for sexual reproduction of multicellular organisms.
    c. Meiosis only occurs in humans. Mitosis only occurs in plants.
    d. Meiosis produces cells that are genetically different. Mitosis produces cells that are genetically identical.

18. Which statement best describes how photosynthesis is different from respiration?
    a. Photosynthesis occurs in animals, but respiration occurs in plants.
    b. During photosynthesis, oxygen is given off, but during respiration, oxygen is taken in.
    c. Photosynthesis requires oxygen, but respiration requires carbon dioxide.
    d. Photosynthesis uses darkness, but respiration uses sunlight.

19. How does the structure of RNA differ from the structure of DNA?
    a. RNA contains 4 nucleotides while DNA contains 6 nucleotides.
    b. RNA contains a double helix while DNA contains a single helix.
    c. RNA contains a single helix while DNA contains a double helix.
    d. The structure of RNA is exactly the same as the structure of DNA.

20. Which type of cell must mutate in order to change an organism's offspring?
    a. Germ cell
    b. Marrow cell
    c. Tissue cell
    d. Ovarian cell

21. How does RNA work with DNA during cell replication?
    a. RNA primes DNA to triple so that daughter cells will have an abundance of DNA material.
    b. DNA primes RNA to triple so that daughter cells will have an abundance of RNA material.
    c. DNA primes RNA replication so that daughter cells will have the same amount of RNA as the parent cell.
    d. RNA primes DNA replication so that daughter cells will have the same amount of DNA as the parent cell.

22. What functions do genes serve in the relationship between parents and offspring?
    a. Genes enable hereditary information to be passed from parents to offspring.
    b. Genes prohibit hereditary information from being passed from parents to offspring.
    c. Genes enable environmental factors to affect parents and offspring.
    d. Genes serve no function in the relationship between parents and offspring.

23. Which statement best describes the structural relationships among chromosomes, genes, and DNA?
    a. A chromosome contains the four genes that make up the DNA double helix.
    b. A gene contains many chromosomes that make up DNA.
    c. A chromosome is a single piece of DNA that contains many genes.
    d. Chromosomes, genes, and DNA have no structural relationships.

24. What does the phenotype describe about an individual?
    a. The phenotype describes a person's genetic makeup.
    b. The phenotype describes a person's observable characteristics.
    c. The phenotype describes a person's environmental factors.
    d. The phenotype describes all the phenomena a person has experienced since birth.

A person with the *T* gene will be tall and a person with the *S* gene will be short. A person with the *B* gene will have black hair and a person with the *R* gene will have red hair. Now consider the Punnett square below.

	T	S
R	Possibility 1	Possibility 2
B	Possibility 3	Possibility 4

The next two questions are based on the information above.

25. What are the characteristics of the person with genes from possibility 1?
    a. Short with black hair
    b. Short with red hair
    c. Tall with black hair
    d. Tall with red hair

26. Which possibility would produce a short offspring with black hair?
    a. Possibility 1
    b. Possibility 2
    c. Possibility 3
    d. Possibility 4

27. Which of the following statements about the sun is FALSE?
    a. The sun is a major external source of heat for Earth.
    b. The sun is a major external source of light for Earth.
    c. The sun is only a minor source of light for Earth since a lot of Earth's light comes from the moon.
    d. Energy from the sun can be used for solar power.

28. Which of the following is an example of an oxidation-reduction (redox) reaction?
    a. Copper loses 2 electrons and silver loses 4 electrons.
    b. Copper loses 2 electrons and silver gains 2 electrons.
    c. Copper gains 2 electrons and silver loses 2 protons.
    d. Copper gains 2 neutrons and silver loses 2 protons.

29. A chemist wants to increase the rate of a reaction between two chemicals. What should he add to the reaction to increase the rate?
    a. A catalyst
    b. An acid
    c. A base
    d. A neutralizer

30. Fill in the blanks in this sentence: Enzymes are _____ molecules that serve as _____ for certain biological reactions.

    a. Enzymes are irrelevant molecules that serve as suppressors for certain biological reactions.

    b. Enzymes are acidic molecules that serve as catalysts for certain biological reactions.

    c. Enzymes are lipid molecules that serve as catalysts for certain biological reactions.

    d. Enzymes are protein molecules that serve as catalysts for certain biological reactions.

31. A lab technician wants to identify an unknown substance. A litmus paper test reveals the pH of the substance is 2. What type of substance is this?

    a. Carcinogen

    b. Water

    c. Acid

    d. Base

32. What type of chemical bond connects the oxygen and hydrogen atoms in a molecule of water?

    a. Static bond

    b. Aquatic bond

    c. Ionic bond

    d. Covalent bond

33. Which of the following statements describes a chemical property of water?

    a. Water has a pH of 1.

    b. A water molecule contains 2 hydrogen atoms and 1 oxygen atom.

    c. A water molecule contains 2 oxygen atoms and 1 hydrogen atom.

    d. The chemical formula for water is HO_2.

34. A man swings a golf club using the following steps:

Step 1: He raises the golf club above his shoulder and stops with club held in midair.

Step 2: He rapids lowers the golf club.

Step 3: He hits the golf ball.

At which step in the swing does the golf club have the most potential energy?

    a. Step 1

    b. Step 2

    c. Step 3

    d. The potential energy is the same at all steps.

35. An atom has 2 protons, 4 neutrons, and 2 electrons. What is the approximate atomic mass of this atom?

    a. 2

    b. 4

    c. 6

    d. 8

36. What are the three major components of an atom?
    a. Positrons, negatrons, and decepticons
    b. Protons, neutrons, and electrons
    c. Molecules, dipoles, and bonds
    d. Proteins, dipoles, and lipids

37. What type of bond is formed when electrons are transferred between atoms?
    a. Transfer bond
    b. Static bond
    c. Covalent bond
    d. Ionic bond

38. The table below contains information from the periodic table of elements.

Element	Atomic number	Approximate atomic weight
B	5	11
C	6	12
N	7	14
O	8	16

Which pattern below best describes the masses of the elements listed in the table?
    a. The elements are listed in random order, C being the heaviest element and N being the lightest element.
    b. The elements are listed in decreasing order, B being the heaviest element and O being the lightest element.
    c. The elements are listed in increasing order, B being the lightest element and O being the heaviest element.
    d. All the elements weigh the same, so the order is irrelevant.

39. Which of the following statements best describes the similarities between gases and liquids?
    a. Gases and liquids both take on the shape of their container.
    b. Gases and liquids both have a fixed shape.
    c. Atoms in a gas and atoms in a liquid are both lighter than air molecules.
    d. Gases have no similarities with liquids.

40. Which statement below best describes the process of condensation?
    a. Condensation is the process of changing from a gas to a liquid.
    b. Condensation is the process of changing from a liquid to a gas.
    c. Condensation is the process of changing from a solid to a liquid.
    d. Condensation is the process of changing from a solid to a gas.

41. A researcher is conducting a survey on the connections between smoking and premature aging. Which of the following questions should the researcher ask survey participants?

    a. Do you enjoy taking surveys?

    b. Are you married?

    c. Do you exercise?

    d. Do you smoke?

42. An organization wants to improve communication between children who are adopted and their biological families. The organization also wants to protect everyone's privacy. Which method below would most improve communication between these two parties?

    a. Create a large book with names, addresses, and other personal information so that adopted children can search for their biological families.

    b. Establish a secure Internet site that helps match adopted children with their biological families.

    c. Publish information in the newspaper about adopted children and their biological families so that people who read the paper can communicate with each other.

    d. Use word of mouth communication so that adopted children can pass messages to their biological families.

43. Every child in a certain family suffers from autism. Based on this evidence, what possible conclusion can be drawn about autism?

    a. Autism may be lethal.

    b. Autism may be genetic.

    c. Autism may be wonderful.

    d. No conclusion can be drawn based on this evidence.

44. Women were more likely to die in childbirth in the 18th century than in the 21st century. What is a possible explanation for why women are less likely to die in childbirth in the present age?

    a. Doctors are better equipped to perform cesarean sections.

    b. Doctors have more tools to monitor mothers during childbirth, so complications can be detected much earlier.

    c. Doctors wash their hands well to avoid transferring germs and infections.

    d. All of the statements above offer reasonable explanations for decreases in mortality during childbirth.

45. A dietician wants to convince a patient to lose weight. Which statement below best communicates a scientific argument that justifies the need for weight loss?

    a. Losing weight can lower blood pressure, increase energy level, and promote overall health.

    b. Society tends to treat overweight people unfairly.

    c. Members of the opposite sex are more interested in people who maintain a healthy weight.

    d. Losing weight is easy to do.

46. A researcher wants to investigate the relationship between family income and quality of medical care. Which statement provides the best reason to conduct this investigation?
    a. The researcher can learn more about wealthy people and ask them for money.
    b. The investigation can help target healthy people so that they can remain healthy.
    c. Results of this investigation may identify a group of people who do not receive quality medical care so that these people could receive better medical treatments.
    d. There is no reason to conduct this investigation.

47. Which of the following statements provides the best reason to include mathematics in scientific research?
    a. Mathematics allows researchers to take an emotional approach to data analysis.
    b. Mathematics allows researchers to take an objective approach to data analysis.
    c. Mathematics allows researchers to take an unrealistic approach to data analysis.
    d. Mathematics allows researchers to take an artistic approach to data analysis.

48. All of the following statements are reasons to include technology in scientific research EXCEPT:
    a. Technology can allow researchers to access a large number of research participants.
    b. Technology can allow researchers to fabricate research results.
    c. Technology can allow researchers to analyze a large amount of data.
    d. Technology can allow researchers to conduct a wide variety of different experiments.

49. What is the name for the reactant that is entirely consumed by the reaction?
    a. limiting reactant
    b. reducing agent
    c. reaction intermediate
    d. reagent

50. What is the name for the horizontal rows of the periodic table?
    a. groups
    b. periods
    c. families
    d. sets

51. What is the mass (in grams) of 7.35 mol water?
    a. 10.7 g
    b. 18 g
    c. 132 g
    d. 180.6 g

52. What is 119°K in degrees Celsius?
    a. 32°C
    b. –154°C
    c. 154°C
    d. –32°C

53. How many different types of tissue are there in the human body?
    a. four
    b. six
    c. eight
    d. ten

54. What is the name of the outermost layer of skin?
    a. dermis
    b. epidermis
    c. subcutaneous tissue
    d. hypodermis

Section 4. English and Language Usage	Number of Questions: **34**
	Time Limit: **34 Minutes**

1. The Declaration of Independence contains these famous lines: "When in the Course of human events it becomes necessary for one people to dissolve the political bands which have connected them with another...a decent respect to the opinions of mankind requires that they should declare the causes which impel them to the separation." Which of the following best explains the purpose of the ellipses in the passage?
   a. to indicate emphasis
   b. to indicate excluded material
   c. to indicate quoted material
   d. to indicate more than one point of view

2. The soldier was awarded the ____ for his display of courage, strength, and ____ in battle. Which of the following words correctly completes the sentence?
   a. metal; mettle
   b. medal; metal
   c. medal; mettle
   d. mettle; metal

3. The teacher reminded the class that each student was responsible for ____ work and that any cheating or plagiarizing would be swiftly punished. Which of the following correctly completes the sentence?
   a. their
   b. his
   c. his or her
   d. ones

4. Thomas Macaulay once commented that "Few of the many wise *apothegms* which have been uttered have prevented a single foolish action." Which of the following best explains the meaning of *apothegms* as it is used in the sentence?
   a. advice
   b. preferences
   c. quotes
   d. sayings

5. A childhood reading of *Tales from Shakespeare* permanently ____ Helene's interest in studying the Great Bard. Which of the following correctly completes the sentence?
   a. piqued
   b. peaked
   c. peked
   d. peeked

6. Which of the following demonstrates correct punctuation?
    a. Graham still needs the following items for his class: a sable brush, soft pastels, a sketchbook, and an easel.
    b. Graham still needs the following items for his class, a sable brush, soft pastels, a sketchbook, and an easel.
    c. Graham still needs the following items for his class: a sable brush; soft pastels; a sketchbook; and an easel.
    d. Graham still needs the following items for his class – a sable brush; soft pastels; a sketchbook; and an easel.

7. The French and Indian War was not an isolated war in North America. It was part of a larger war that Europe was fighting. Europeans called it the Seven Years' War. Which of the following options best combines the sentence? Consider style, clarity, and conciseness when choosing your response.
    a. The French and Indian War did not occur in North America but was rather a small part of the larger European war known as the Seven Years' War.
    b. What Europeans called the Seven Years' War was called the French and Indian War in North America. It was part of a larger war that Europe was fighting.
    c. The French and Indian War was not an isolated war in North America but was rather part of a larger war that Europe was fighting, known among Europeans as the Seven Years' War.
    d. While North America was fighting the French and Indian War, the Europeans were fighting a much larger war known as the Seven Years' War.

8. During the Seven Years' War, England and France fought over the control of the North American colonies, as well as the trade routes to those colonies. Which of the following words functions as a verb in the sentence above?
    a. fought
    b. control
    c. trade
    d. those

9. Which of the following is a simple sentence?
    a. Following the French and Indian War, Spain gave up Florida to England.
    b. England returned part of Cuba to Spain, while France gave up part of Louisiana.
    c. France lost most of its Caribbean islands, and England gained dominance over them.
    d. Because every nation lost something, no clear victor was declared.

10. Which of the following sentences follows the rules of capitalization?
    a. One major conflict in the Seven Years' War occurred between the Prussian Hohenzollern Family and the Austrian Hapsburg Family.
    b. The Hapsburg family was considered to be the rulers of the Holy Roman empire.
    c. At the start of the war, Maria Theresa was the empress of Austria and was strengthening Austria's military.
    d. Frederick the Great of Prussia had recently acquired the former Austrian Province of Silesia.

11. Which of the following sentences demonstrates the correct use of quotation marks?
    a. Maria Theresa was the mother of Marie Antoinette, the French queen remembered for saying, 'Let them eat cake.'
    b. Maria Theresa was the mother of Marie Antoinette, the French queen remembered for saying, 'Let them eat cake'.
    c. Maria Theresa was the mother of Marie Antoinette, the French queen remembered for saying, "Let them eat cake."
    d. Maria Theresa was the mother of Marie Antoinette, the French queen remembered for saying, "Let them eat cake".

12. Which of the following sentences contains a correct example of subject-verb agreement?
    a. Some of the post-rally fervor have already died down.
    b. Gary, as well as his three children, are coming to visit later today.
    c. Are neither Robert nor his parents planning to see the presentation?
    d. We waited patiently while a herd of moose was crossing the mountain highway.

13. I tried to call Lisle earlier, but I could not get her on the phone. Which of the following words functions as an adverb in the sentence?
    a. call
    b. earlier
    c. could
    d. phone

14. The Hapsburg rule of the Austro-Hungarian Empire effectively ended with the reign of Franz Joseph I (1848-1916). Which of the following best explains the purpose of the parentheses in the sentence above?
    a. to indicate the page numbers in the book where this information might be found
    b. to tell the reader when the Austro-Hungarian empire collapsed
    c. to identify information that was located using another source
    d. to set off useful information that does not fit directly into the flow of the sentence

15. Which of the following sentences is grammatically correct?
    a. The person who left the trash in the hallway needs to pick it up now.
    b. Nobody needs to turn in their projects before the end of the month.
    c. Every new instructor should stop by the main office to pick up his room key.
    d. Both Simeon and Ruth are generous with his or her time.

16. I never know when you are joking about something. What is the point of view indicated by the underlined words in the sentence above?
    a. third; second
    b. second; first
    c. first; second
    d. first; third

17. Maud will try to be there by 4:00, but she will _____ be there no later than 4.30. Which of the following correctly completes the sentence?
    a. defiantly
    b. definitely
    c. defanately
    d. definetly

18. "*Walking* is a very good exercise that the majority of people can incorporate into their daily lives." A verbal is a verb form that is used as a different part of speech. In the above sentence, which part of speech is the word *walking* used as?
    a. noun
    b. adverb
    c. adjective
    d. conjunction

19. In the fairy tale *Sleeping Beauty*, the story opens with the christening of a princess. All of the fairies are invited except one; and when this one fairy realizes that she has been overlooked, she utters a *malediction* upon the princess that results in the princess pricking her finger on a spindle and falling asleep for one hundred years. Which of the following best explains the meaning of *malediction* as it is used in the passage?
    a. enchantment
    b. remedy
    c. promise
    d. curse

20. The story of *Sleeping Beauty* is similar to many fairy tales. Its origins are unknown. It is believed to be a combination of different versions of an old story. One of the most familiar versions comes from the French collection of fairy tales by Charles Perrault. The German Brothers Grimm also incorporated elements into their publication.

Which of the following options best combines the sentences above without losing the meaning of the passage? Consider style and clarity when choosing a response.
    a. The story of *Sleeping Beauty* is similar to many fairy tales, because its origins are unknown. It is believed to be a combination of different versions of an old story. One of the most familiar versions comes from the French collection of fairy tales by Charles Perrault. The German Brothers Grimm also incorporated elements into their publication.
    b. The origins of *Sleeping Beauty* are unknown, but like many fairy tales it is believed to be a combination of different versions of an old story. The most familiar version is that of the French Charles Perrault. Another familiar version comes from the German Brothers Grimm.
    c. Like many fairy tales, the origins of *Sleeping Beauty* are unknown, and it is believed to be a combination of different versions of an old story. One of the most familiar versions comes from the French collection of fairy tales by Charles Perrault, while the German Brothers Grimm also incorporated elements into their publication.
    d. One of the most familiar versions of *Sleeping Beauty* comes from the French collection of fairy tales by Charles Perrault, and the German Brothers Grimm also incorporated elements into their publication. But the story of *Sleeping Beauty* is similar to that of many fairy tales. Its origins are unknown, and it is believed to be a combination of different versions of an old story.

21. Which of the following sentences demonstrates the correct use of an apostrophe?
   a. In one version of the story, there are seven fairy's invited to the christening, while in another version there are twelve fairy's.
   b. Some historians' believe that the number twelve represents the shift from a lunar year of thirteen months to a solar year of twelve months.
   c. Other historians claim that the symbolism in the fairy tale is more about nature and the shifting season's.
   d. Regardless of its meaning, the fairy tale remains popular and has been immortalized in Tchaikovsky's music for the ballet.

22. The teacher spoke firmly to the class: "If <u>you</u> want to succeed in this course, be willing to work hard and turn in work on time." Which of the following points of view is indicated by the underlined word in the above sentence?
   a. first-person singular
   b. third-person plural
   c. second-person plural
   d. third-person singular

23. Which of the following is not a simple sentence?
   a. Agatha Christie was the author of more than sixty detective novels.
   b. Her most famous detectives were Hercule Poirot and Miss Marple.
   c. She also wrote over fifteen collections of short stories about these detectives.
   d. Most readers favor Poirot, but Christie preferred Miss Marple.

24. Hercule Poirot is remembered not only for his genius in solving mysteries, but also for his *fastidious* habits and his commitment to personal grooming. Which of the following best explains the meaning of *fastidious* as it is used in the sentence?
   a. fussy
   b. lazy
   c. old-fashioned
   d. hilarious

25. The elderly Miss Marple, on the other hand, is remembered for solving the mysteries she encounters by making seemingly *extraneous* connections to life in her small village. Which of the following best explains the meaning of *extraneous* as it is used in the sentence?
   a. sophisticated
   b. irrelevant
   c. diligent
   d. useful

26. At a party, Thornton is usually the first one on the dance floor, but unfortunately he has no ____.
Which of the following correctly completes the sentence?
    a. rhythym
    b. rythym
    c. rhthym
    d. rhythm

27. In *Modern American Usage*, Wilson Follett noted the following example of a dangling modifier:
"Leaping to the saddle, his horse bolted." Which of the following sentences removes the dangling
modifier from the above sentence while retaining style and clarity?
    a. His horse bolted as it leaped to the saddle.
    b. When he leaped to the saddle, his horse bolted.
    c. His horse bolting, he leaped to the saddle.
    d. He leaped to the saddle, his horse bolted.

28. You'll have to ask Hilda; the choice is ____. Which of the following correctly completes the
sentence?
    a. hers
    b. her's
    c. hers'
    d. hers's

29. The word *anaesthetic* refers to medication that causes a temporary loss of feeling or sensation.
This word is made up of two primary Greek parts: the root *aesthet* and the prefix *an-*. The root word
aesthet means "feeling." Based on the meaning of the word in medical usage, which is the most
likely meaning of the prefix *an-*?
    a. without
    b. against
    c. away
    d. before

30. The years leading up to the American Civil War are often referred to using the term *antebellum*.
This word is composed of two primary Latin parts: the root *bellum*, which means "war," and the
prefix *ante-*. Based on the contextual usage of this word, what is the most likely meaning of the
prefix *ante-*?
    a. again
    b. good
    c. before
    d. together

31. _____ went to the movies after having dinner at Lenny's.
    a. Her and I
    b. Her and me
    c. She and I
    d. She and me

32. Which word is *not* spelled correctly in the context of the following sentence?
Dr. Vargas was surprised that the prescription had effected Ron's fatigue so dramatically.
    a. surprised
    b. prescription
    c. effected
    d. fatigue

33. Which word is *not* spelled correctly in the context of the following sentence?
The climate hear is inappropriate for snow sports such as skiing.
    a. climate
    b. hear
    c. inappropriate
    d. skiing

34. Which word is *not* used correctly in the context of the following sentence?
Before you walk any further, beware of the approaching traffic.
    a. before
    b. further
    c. beware
    d. approaching

Answer Explanations

Reading Answer Explanations

1. C: The best starting point for a research project on the Globe Theatre of London would be the Encyclopedia Britannica. A thesaurus is an excellent place to find synonyms, while a dictionary is an excellent place to find word meanings. However, neither would contain information about the history of the Globe Theatre. (While writing, Ernestine might find herself in need of a better word or a word meaning; in this case, the thesaurus and dictionary will be useful.) A Latin dictionary would not be useful for researching the history of the Globe Theatre.

2. B: The student does not have to be familiar with the Romance languages to know that "American" is a nationality, not a language. (The primary language spoken in America is usually considered to be English.) Based on this information alone, choice B can be selected as the correct answer. The other languages listed in the answer choices (Spanish, French, and Portuguese) are both recognized languages and Romance languages.

3. A: The word *consonantal* would fall between the words *considerable* and *conspicuous* on a dictionary page. The word *consumption* would follow *conspicuous*, while the words *conserve* and *conquistador* would precede *considerable*.

4. C: Of the answer choices given, the word that would most likely appear on the previous dictionary page is *conserve*, which is alphabetically closer to *considerable* than *conquistador* is. Both *considerable* and *conserve* begin with *cons-*. The vowel that follows is different. The word *conquistador*, however, has only *con-* in common with *considerable*. This leaves far more room for words (and potentially pages) in between these two entries. The word *consonantal* would fall between the words *considerable* and *conspicuous* on a dictionary page. The word *consumption* would follow *conspicuous*.

5. C: The best synonym is *abundance*, which suggests that Kit has more zucchini than she needs, and is therefore trying to offload zucchini on anyone who might want some. The *plethora* might lead to a mild *irritation*, but the words are definitely not synonyms. (In some cases, a *plethora* is certainly not an irritation.) The word *plethora* is related to a *quantity*, but it is a specific type of quantity: an excess. Because the word *quantity* can also describe a lack of something, these words are not synonyms. Kit is obviously trying to avoid *waste*, but the words *plethora* and *waste* are not synonyms. *Waste* would also not be a natural replacement for *plethora* in the sentence.

6. B: When the directions are followed correctly, the new word is REVERT. The words REVEST and REVERSE require the addition of an S. (REVERSE also requires a second E.) The word REVIEW requires the addition of an I (which has been removed) and a W.

7. B: If Ethan buys his pens from Office in Bulk, he will pay $450 for 500 pens. At Specialty Pens, he would pay $485; at Office Warehouse, he would pay $475; at Ballpoint & Lead, he would pay $495.

8. D: The symbol /\ appears numerous times on the map, so the best way to determine the actual number of mountain ranges is to use the text on the map. In the state of Wyoming, six separate ranges are identified: the Wyoming Range, the Teton Range, the Wind River Range, the Bighorn Mountains, the Rocky Mountains (which are part of a much larger mountain range that crosses a number of states), and the Laramie Mountains. All of the other answer choices identify too few ranges. (From a purely technical perspective, all of these smaller ranges are actually part of the larger range of Rocky Mountains that shapes this part of the United States. Because the map identifies the separate ranges, however, it is accurate to recognize the distinctions. What is more, there is nothing on the map to indicate that all of these ranges are part of the Rockies, so the test taker may count each one separately.)

9. B: On the map, the star symbol is underneath the city of Cheyenne, which is the capital. The other answer choices – Laramie, Jackson, and Sheridan – are not identified as the capital city.

10. A: Two national parks are identified on the map: Grand Teton National Park and Yellowstone National Park. There is also a national monument (Devils Tower National Monument), but since the question says nothing about national monuments and specifies national *parks*, answer choice B can be ruled out. Choices C and D are too high.

11. B: Colorado and Utah lie along Wyoming's southern border. Idaho lies to the west; Nebraska and South Dakota lie to the east; Montana lies along the northern border.

12. D: If Beryl knew something instinctively, it is safe to say that her mother's warning was not stated outright. Therefore, answer choice D is the best option. Answer choice A makes little sense. Answer choice B makes sense only if Beryl suspects her mother does not care whether or not she smokes. Answer choice C has a meaning that is the opposite of the one implied in the sentence.

13. C: The passage is expository, because it *exposes* or reveals information about the topic. A narrative passage tells a story; this passage does not. A technical passage provides the reader with instructions or details about completing a certain activity; this passage does not. A persuasive passage attempts to convince the reader to agree with the author's viewpoint about a topic. There is nothing persuasive about this passage.

14. B: Answer choice B, the second-to-last sentence in the passage, best summarizes the main point of the passage: that although The Five might not have had solid formal training, they influenced Russian music, and that influence extended beyond their own era. Answer choice A is too specific, and focuses on those who were influenced rather than on the actual composers who made up The Five. Because it is the opening sentence of the passage, answer choice C is a good option. However, answer choice B gets more to the heart of the topic. Answer choice C leaves out the information about long-term influence, so it is not the best option for a summary sentence. Answer choice D focuses on only two of The Five, so it cannot be a summary statement for the entire passage.

15. C: The final two sentences of the passage suggest that answer C is the best choice: "Composers such as Alexander Glazunov, Sergei Prokofiev, and Igor Stravinsky studied under Rimsky-Korsakov. Additionally, the mid-twentieth century composer Dmitri Shostakovich studied under Glazunov, creating a legacy of musical understanding that persisted well beyond the era of The Five." While the author does not explicitly state that Rimsky-Korsakov was the most influential, he is the only composer who is specifically linked to later composers. These noted composers include Rimsky-Korsakov's own students (Glazunov, Prokofiev, and Stravinsky) and one of his student's students (Shostakovich). Based on this, it is reasonable to conclude that the author would agree that Rimsky-Korsakov was the most influential of "The Five." While the other individuals listed in the answer choices had a definite influence on music and composed notable works, none of them is specifically linked to later composers in the passage.

16. D: The symbol that divides the word *collar* in half indicates the syllables, which in this case are *col* and *lar*. The symbol cannot indicate emphasis, because the word is simply divided in half. The spelling of the word is clear by looking at it, so there is no need to split the word in half to indicate spelling. And while origin is indicated later in the dictionary entry, there is nothing about the initial presentation of the word to suggest that the symbol in the middle indicates the word's origin.

17. A: The bold font indicates that the first part of the word is emphasized when the word is pronounced: **col**-lar instead of col-**lar**. A bold font is almost never a part of a word's spelling (except perhaps in the spelling of words for businesses), so there is no need to bold any part of the word to indicate spelling. The bold font does nothing to indicate the word's origin. While the bold font does appear in one part of the word and not the other, this does not in itself indicate the syllables in the way the symbol between the two halves of the word does. For instance, the word could be written **col**lar, and this would still suggest emphasis rather than indicate the word's syllables.

18. D: The earliest word in the information about the word's origin is *collum*. All other origins appear to date back to this word. *Collum*, which led to a Latin word (*collare*), led to the Old French form *colier*, which eventually became the Middle English form *coler*. This later evolved into the Modern English word *collar*. The earliest language origin indicated is Latin.

19. C: Since the crime is fairly obvious, Ena is surprised that the child's lie is so *shameless*. Answer choice A is incorrect, because there is nothing *effective* about the child's lie. The child may be *arrogant* in assuming he will get away with lying, but this option is not as strong as answer choice C. There is nothing in the sentence to suggest that the child's lie is *hostile*, so answer choice D makes little sense.

20. D: The heading notes that the information is related to *monarchs* within the *Stuart* family. There are two significant problems with Oliver Cromwell being included in this list: (1) he is not a Stuart (since his last name is Cromwell), and (2) he is identified as a "lord protector" instead of someone who reigned in England. The test taker does not have to be familiar with English history to spot this anomaly. All of the other answer choices are reigning monarchs of the Stuart family.

21. B: The reign of Charles I ended in 1649. Between 1653 and 1658, Oliver Cromwell is noted as "lord protector," and then there is another break of two years before Charles II assumes the throne in 1660. Additionally, James II's reign ends in 1688, but Mary II does not assume the throne until 1689. For all of the other monarchs listed (except Charles II), the starting date of their reign coincides with the ending date of the previous monarch's reign, so this break – albeit brief – is still considered a break. (Historically, James II was forced to abdicate in late December of 1688 after what many believed to be the faked birth of a male heir, and his daughter, Mary, did not take over for a few weeks after this. She ruled alongside her husband, William III. This was truly a short break in the monarchy, but it was definitely a break. It represented a period during which England was without a recognized monarch.)

22. C: Throughout the passage, the author compares and contrasts the Arthurian writings of Malory and Tennyson, so the structure of the passage is clearly comparison-contrast. No problem is presented, so no solution must be posited. A passage written using a sequence structure would be focused on presenting information for the reader to follow in order (i.e. a "how-to" essay). The author essentially goes back and forth between Malory and Tennyson, so this passage does not employ a sequence structure. While there are some statements indicating cause and effect – Tennyson is said to have been influenced by Malory, for instance – the focus of the passage is more on comparing the two authors.

23. D: The following differences between Malory and Tennyson are noted in the passage: 1) Malory wrote in prose, while Tennyson wrote in poetry. 2) Malory wrote during the Medieval era, while Tennyson wrote during the Victorian era. 3) Malory was more focused on heroism and morality, while Tennyson was more focused on nature and elegy. The author of the passage mentions that Malory wrote about Gareth, Tristan, and Isolde, but there is not enough information in the passage to argue that Tennyson did *not*.

24. D: The passage is primarily about Malory and Tennyson. The author includes useful information toward the end of the passage to indicate what Tennyson's contemporary influences might have been (that is, "social problems and the need for social justice" within his own era). The information about Charles Dickens, however, seems to come out of nowhere. It does not merit a place in the passage, since the author says nothing about a similar author in Malory's time, which would make the comparison complete. As a result, the information about Dickens is irrelevant. The other answer choices, however, contain useful information that develops the author's main point.

25. A: In the first paragraph, the author notes that Malory was a Medieval writer who "focused more on the moral elements within these stories." This statement would also be true of Medieval literature in general. In the second paragraph, the author says that it has been argued that Tennyson "was writing an allegory about social problems and the need for social justice that existed during Tennyson's own time." This writing would also reflect the interests and defining qualities of the author's era. Therefore, answer choice A is correct. The author of the passage compares and contrasts the two writers' works, but there is nothing in the passage to suggest that he or she is taking a stand on which writer's work is superior. As a result, answer choices B and C are incorrect. Answer choice D counters the information at the start of the second paragraph that says Tennyson was "heavily influenced" by Malory. Even though Tennyson might have put his own spin on the Arthurian legends, he was still clearly influenced by Malory.

26. B: Without seeing an ingredient list for each soup, the best the test taker can do is look at the names and determine whether or not any form of dairy is likely included in the soup. Egg is a type of dairy, so the egg drop soup is not a good option for Regina. Additionally, the cheese in the broccoli cheese soup and the cream in the cream of tomato soup are likely to be problematic for Regina. No dairy products are listed in "lentil soup," so this may be assumed to be the safest choice. (In traditional Mediterranean and Middle Eastern preparation, lentil soup does not typically include dairy products.)

27. C: The final column in the chart indicates the percentage of each country's population that was lost. For Romania, this percentage is 9.33. The percentages for the other choices are half of this or less. Of the nations listed in the chart, Romania certainly fared the worst in terms of the percentage of the population that was lost, even if the actual numbers are lower than they are for other nations.

28. C: Looking only at the numbers, the casualties in Russia are staggeringly high: 2,254,369 military deaths, 4,950,000 military wounded, and 1,500,000 civilian deaths. The fact that these numbers represent only 2.14 percent of Russia's population speaks to how many people were in Russia at the time. (According to the chart, the total population was 175,100,000.) The casualty numbers for the United Kingdom are also high, but nowhere near as high as they are for Russia. The numbers for Belgium and Romania are also high. In Romania, these losses represent a large percentage of the population. Russia, however, suffered the highest number of casualties, which is the focus of the question.

29. C: In Romania, civilian deaths are listed at 450,000. This represents 6 percent of the total population of 7,500,000. The civilian deaths in Belgium represent less than 1 percent of the total population. This is also true for Russia, despite the higher actual number of deaths. In Italy, civilian deaths represent a little over 1.5 percent of the population, which is still far below the percentage for Romania.

30. D: The chart notes that civilian deaths are ones that are due to war, famine, and disease. Answer choice A is certainly related to war. However, the sinking of the RMS *Lusitania*, while tragic and certainly a cause of civilian deaths, would not have caused such a large number of casualties. Answer choices B and C reference events that seem exclusive to the battlefield: the trench warfare system and the mustard gas used on the battlefield. While civilians were certainly affected by these events, these answer choices seem to exclude civilian involvement. Both specifically mention battlefield activity. If an answer choice had mentioned the bombing or gassing of towns, however, this would have suggested civilian involvement. The Spanish Influenza epidemic is the most logical choice, in large part because it fits the "disease" category very well. The fact that the epidemic struck Europe at the end of the war (note the dates of the war that are included at the top of the chart) and affected what must have been an already weakened population makes this event a likely cause of a significant number of civilian deaths during World War I.

31. C: The announcement includes the following sentence: "To offset the crowding, the university has polled the various departments about schedules, and has settled on a recommended roster for when the members of each department should visit the faculty canteen for lunch." This suggests that the university made every effort to find out the schedules for each department and create a lunch arrangement that would give the members of each department the best opportunity possible to visit the canteen. The list is clearly not arranged alphabetically, so answer choice A is incorrect. The university definitely contacted the departments, as noted in the announcement. However, since the announcement mentions respecting the schedule and says nothing about an approval process, it is difficult to determine whether or not the university is worried about whether the faculty members will be amenable to the new lunch roster. Therefore, answer choice B can be eliminated. Finally, answer choice D seems to contradict the information in the announcement, so it too is incorrect. If the university contacted the departments about faculty schedules, the university obviously put some thought into the schedule. Answer choice D would suggest an arbitrary decision about scheduling, with no thought given to current faculty department schedules.

32. B: The final two sentences are as follows: "We ask that all faculty members respect this schedule. Faculty will be expected to display a department badge before entering the canteen for lunch." The overall recommendation is that faculty members should honor the schedule, with the added implication that faculty members will either not be allowed to enter the canteen outside of the posted lunch roster or that departments will be notified if the faculty members do make this effort. No doubt the announcement is also a recommendation to bring the badge, but there is an undercurrent of warning in it that goes beyond a "friendly reminder." Therefore, answer choice A is incorrect. There is nothing in the announcement or in the two final sentences to suggest that the university wants faculty members to eat lunch elsewhere, so answer choice C is incorrect. Answer choice D is a good option, but it infers just a little too much from the final two sentences. While university sanctions might very well be imposed on faculty members who don't follow the schedule, these two sentences alone are simply a word of caution to faculty members that the schedule needs to be respected. Answer choice D goes too far, so it too is incorrect.

33. C: Angela's reading list appears to consist of classic works of literature, as the opening statement notes that she "read the following classics." This means that "The Cask of Amontillado" by Edgar Allen Poe is unlikely to be a newspaper article, a book chapter by itself that is separate from the rest of the book, or a television show episode. Based on the information provided, it is most likely a short story.

34. A: The italics indicate full-length published books. The italics cannot represent works of classic literature. This is because according to the sentence, "The Cask of Amontillado" is also a classic. However, it is not italicized. Similarly, the italics cannot represent Angela's summer reading or the books that she has completed, because the item in quotation marks is also on Angela's summer reading list. (Additionally, in the case of answer choice D, the sentence states that Angela "read" these works, so the sentence itself indicates they have all been completed.)

35. B: If the student's nerves are getting the better of him, it is likely that he is either very pale or very flushed. Because *flushed* is one of the options, it is the correct choice. A complexion cannot be *rambling*, so answer choice A is incorrect. Answer choice C has a hint of promise, but it makes the sentence more confusing, so it too is incorrect. It is difficult to know what is meant by the phrase "*weak* complexion," so answer choice D is too unclear to be correct.

36. D: Even if the test taker is unfamiliar with the meaning of *puerile*, the word *fantasies* should suggest something childish. The overall tone indicates an attitude of distaste toward the book. Consider the following wording in particular: "most likely to be enjoyed only by those with puerile fantasies." *Only* limits the audience, and *puerile fantasies* limits it even further. Answer choice A is incorrect, because the author makes no recommendations, and comments only on who might enjoy the book. Answer choice B is possible, but the tone would suggest that the *puerile fantasies* are not so much natural (as an appreciation for fantasy literature would be to children), but rather unique to a limited audience of adults. Answer choice C is incorrect, because the overall implication of the statement is that the book will appeal to a very limited audience. This leaves answer choice D, which is the best option: the author of the review believes the book would not appeal to mature adults.

37. A: Only Twin Theatres does not have a showing before 6 p.m. or after 10 p.m. The other cinemas have at least one showing before or after these times.

38. D: The only showing available after 10.30 p.m. is the 11.25 p.m. showing at Best Seat in The House. None of the other cinemas has a showing after 10.30 p.m.

39. B: Residents with addresses ending in 7 may water on Wednesdays, so the Morgan family should set up its watering schedule for this day of the week. The other days are for people with addresses that end in numbers other than 7.

40. C: The final sentence of the announcement notes the following: "Businesses with suite numbers should use the final number in the suite number to determine their watering schedule." No doubt this is due to the fact that businesses with suite numbers will have the same street address as a number of other businesses. Using the suite number will help spread out the watering schedule. In the case of the Everby Title Company, the suite address ends in 3, so the watering day is Thursday. Based on the information in the announcement, the other answer choices can be eliminated.

41. A: There is no explanation regarding the organization of the schedule, nor does the announcement say anything about why there is only one number assigned to Friday and Saturday. The announcement does say that the watering limitations reflect an "effort to conserve water," so the best inference is that the city has found that there are more addresses ending in these numbers (4 and 5), and has therefore adjusted the schedule accordingly. There is no way to determine from the announcement whether or not all businesses end in these numbers, or whether or not businesses consume more water, so answer choice B is incorrect. It is impossible to determine from the announcement if residents at these addresses consume more water, so answer choice C is incorrect. Similarly, there is nothing in the announcement to indicate that the city is more concerned about water usage in the latter part of the week – or why the part of the week would make a difference – so answer choice D is incorrect. The announcement only notes a goal of water conservation, and that water usage will be allotted by address. Therefore, the most logical assumption is that there are more addresses ending in 4 and 5 than in the other numbers.

42. C: Sybilla is clearly trying to improve her financial situation, so the word *strengthen* makes the most sense. The word *add* captures the idea, but it does not fit into the sentence as a synonym for *aggrandize*. The word *develop* has promise, but it does not capture the meaning in the same way as *strengthen* does when used in place of *aggrandize*. The word *dispute* makes no sense in the context of the sentence.

43. C: Since both authors are explaining in the passages how the same story may come to be in different cultures, it is clear they both accept that there are often common elements in fairy tales from different cultures.

44. A: The author of Passage 2 claims that the essence and nature of fairy tales is their representation of basic human experience. It is this assertion that leads the author to believe that the same story could develop independently in different places.

45. D: The author does not mention the movement of food in the passage.

46. B: The author never mentions witches in the passage.

47. A: The passage suggests that spelunking is an outdoorsy, family adventure, then goes on to describe the adventure of going to a cave. If you do not already know that spelunking is another word for caving, you can infer this information based on reading the passage.

48. B: The article's style is not technical or scientific in the least. It is a simple and lighthearted article about something a family could do together. It is adventurous, but *Adventures for Men* is not a good choice since the fun is for the whole family. *Mud Magazine* might have been the next best choice, but *Family Fun Days* is clearly better. Your job is to choose the best choice of the options given.

Mathematics Answer Explanations

1. D: Nurse Andrew had to recommend patients for a study about high blood pressure and high cholesterol. According to the problem statement, $\frac{3}{5}$ of his patients fit this category. Therefore, convert $\frac{3}{5}$ to a percentage using these steps:
$$3 \div 5 = 0.60 \text{ and } (0.60)(100) = 60\%$$

2. A: Dr. Lee noticed that 5% of 30% of his patients were hospitalized. So multiply 30% by 5% using these steps:
Convert 30% and 5% into decimals by dividing both numbers by 100.
$$\frac{30}{100} = 0.30 \text{ and } \frac{5}{100} = 0.05$$
Now multiply 0.30 by 0.05 to get
$$(0.30)(0.05) = 0.015$$
Now convert 0.015 to a percentage by multiplying by 100.
$$(0.015)(100) = 1.5\%$$

3. D: The patient's dosage must increase by 30%. So calculate 30% of 270:
$$(0.30)(270 \text{ mg}) = 81 \text{ mg}$$
Now add the 30% increase to the original dosage.
$$270 \text{ mg} + 81 \text{ mg} = 351 \text{ mg}$$

4. C: Since 60% of the patients in the study were women, 40% of the patients were men. Calculate the number of male patients by multiplying 500 by 0.40.
$$(500)(0.40) = 200$$

Of the 200 male patients in the study, 20% experienced some trauma as a child. So 80% did not experience a childhood trauma. Multiply 200 by 0.80 to get the final answer.

$$(200)(0.80) = 160$$

5. C: If the incoming class has 200 students, then $\frac{1}{2}$ of those students were required to take the exam.

$$(200)\left(\frac{1}{2}\right) = 100$$

So 100 students took the exam but only $\frac{3}{5}$ of that 100 passed the exam.

$$(100)\left(\frac{3}{5}\right) = 60$$

Therefore 60 students passed the exam.

6. B: The first roommate receives $1000 per month, and he uses $\frac{1}{4}$ of that amount for rent and utilities.

$$(\$1000)\left(\frac{1}{4}\right) = \$250$$

So the student pays $250 for rent and utilities, which leaves him with
$$\$1000 - \$250 = \$750$$
The student divides the remaining $750 in half.
$$\frac{\$750}{2} = \$375$$
The student saves $375 and lives off the remaining $375.

7. B: The second roommate budgets $\frac{1}{5}$ of his check for dining out plus another $\frac{1}{4}$ of his check for social activities. So add $\frac{1}{5}$ and $\frac{1}{4}$ by first finding a common denominator.

$$\frac{1}{5} = \frac{4}{20} \text{ and } \frac{1}{4} = \frac{5}{20}$$
$$\frac{4}{20} + \frac{5}{20} = \frac{9}{20}$$

8. D: First add all expenses for the third roommate. Then subtract his total expenses from $1000.
$$\$250 + \$100 + \$25 = \$375$$
$$\$1000 - \$375 = \$625$$

9. A: The ratio of his savings to his rent is 1:3, which means that for every $3 he pays in rent, he saves $1 for the purchase of a house. So to calculate the amount the fourth roommate saves for the purchase of a house, divide $270 by 3.

$$\frac{\$270}{3} = \$90$$

10. C: Each roommate donated about $12 towards the gift purchase.
$$\$12 + \$12 + \$12 = \$36$$

11. A: To obtain the length of the new routine, subtract 7 minutes from the length of the original routine, which was 45 minutes.

$$45 \text{ minutes} - 7 \text{ minutes} = 38 \text{ minutes}$$

12. C: Find $\frac{1}{6}$ of 500 by multiplying

$$(500)\left(\frac{1}{6}\right) = \frac{500}{6} = 83.3333$$

$\frac{500}{6}$ is an improper fraction. Convert the fraction to a decimal and round to the nearest hundredth to get 83.33.

13. D: The Roman numeral system requires adding or subtracting the individual digits in order to obtain the full number. The L equals 50 and X equals 10. So LX means add 50 + 10 to get 60. The I equals 1 and V equals 5. However, since the I is placed directly before the V, subtract 5 − 1 to get 4. Finally, add 60 + 4 to get 64.

14. C: Veronica receives $70,000. First she contributes 15% of her salary to a retirement account.
$$($70,000)(0.15) = 10,500$$
$$$70,000 − $10,500 = $59,500$$
After contributing to her retirement account, Veronica has $59,500 left. Then she pays 30% in taxes.
$$($59,500)(0.30) = $17,850$$
$$$59,500 − $17,850 = $41,650$$
After paying taxes, Veronica has $41,650 left. Finally, she pays $70 each month for health insurance. Calculate the annual amount Veronica pays for health insurance, and subtract this amount from her remaining salary.
$$($70)(12) = $840$$
$$$41,750 − $840 = $40,810$$

15. B: To determine the total cost of Veronica's new car, add all her expenditures.
$$$40,210 + $3,015 + $5,218 = $48,443$$

16. A: The beginning balance for the account was $503.81. Then one deposit was made. So add the amount of that deposit to the beginning balance.
$$$503.81 + 125.00 = $628.81$$
Next, an ATM was used to withdraw money from the account. So subtract the amount of the withdrawal from the new balance.
$$$628.81 − $215.00 = $413.81$$
Finally, add the monthly interest earned to obtain the ending balance.
$$$413.81 + $5.38 = 419.19$$

17. C: Apply the order of operations to solve this problem. Multiplication and division are computed first from left to right. Then addition and subtraction are computed next from left to right.
$$2 + (2)(4) − 4 \div 2 =$$
$$2 + 8 − 4 \div 2 =$$
$$2 + 8 − 2 =$$
$$10 − 2 =$$
$$8$$

18. A: The hospital staff will order 1 pizza for each group of 4 people, and 160 people will attend the event.
$$160 \div 4 = 40$$

Therefore, the staff will order 40 pizzas. Each pizza costs $9.50. Calculate the total cost for pizzas.
$$(40)($9.50) = $380$$

19. D: Compare and order the rational numbers by finding a common denominator for all three fractions. The least common denominator for 3, 12, and 4 is 12. Now convert the fractions with different denominators into fractions with the same denominator.
$$\frac{1}{3} = \frac{4}{12}$$

$$\frac{5}{12} = \frac{5}{12}$$
$$\frac{1}{4} = \frac{3}{12}$$

Now that all three fractions have the same denominator, order them from largest to smallest by comparing the numerators.

$$\frac{5}{12} > \frac{4}{12} > \frac{3}{12}$$

Since $\frac{5}{12}$ of the doctors are in Group Y, this group has the largest number of doctors. The next largest group has $\frac{4}{12}$ of the doctors, which is Group X. The smallest group has $\frac{3}{12}$ of the doctors, which is Group Z.

20. B: Solve the equation for y.

$$\frac{2y}{10} + 5 = 25$$
$$\frac{2y}{10} = 25 - 5$$
$$\frac{2y}{10} = 20$$
$$2y = (20)(10)$$
$$2y = 200$$
$$y = \frac{200}{2}$$
$$y = 100$$

21. C: Subtract the polynomials by subtracting all the like terms, which have the same variable.
$$8x - 5x = 3x$$
$$7y - 4y = 3y$$
$$6z - 3z = 3z$$
Since 3x, 3y, and 3z are all different terms, the final answer is
$$3x + 3y + 3z$$

22. B: During January, Dr. Lewis worked 20 shifts.
$$\text{shifts for January} = 20$$
During February, she worked three times as many shifts as she did during January.
$$\text{shifts for February} = (20)(3)$$
During March, she worked half the number of shifts she worked in February.
$$\text{shifts for March} = (20)(3)\left(\frac{1}{2}\right)$$

23. D: Use the order of operations to solve this problem. Also remember that the absolute value of a number is always positive.
$$|2 - 10| + (2)(10) - 5 =$$
$$|-8| + (2)(10) - 5 =$$
$$8 + 20 - 5 =$$
$$28 - 5 =$$
$$23$$

24. A: Using the table to list the nurse specialties from largest to smallest gives this order: pediatrics, geriatrics, anesthesia, and midwifery. Therefore, pediatrics should represent the largest slice of the circle graph and midwifery should represent the smallest. Only the graph in choice A fits these criteria.

3 TEAS Practice Tests by Exam Review Press

25. B: The bar for midwifery is shortest of the four. Therefore, midwifery is the specialty with the least number of nurses.

26. C: The variables are the objects the graph measures. In this case, the graph measures the nurse specialties and the number of nurses for each specialty. The dependent variable changes with the independent variable. Here, the number of nurses depends on the particular nurse specialty. Therefore, the independent variable is nurse specialties.

27. C: The prefix, centi-, means 100th. In this case,
$$1 \text{ m} = 100 \text{ cm}$$
Therefore,
$$(7)(1 \text{ m}) = (7)(100 \text{ cm})$$
$$7 \text{ m} = (7)(100 \text{ cm})$$
$$7 \text{ m} = 700 \text{ cm}$$

28. B: A human eyelash is one centimeter long. Nanometers are much too short to describe an eyelash. Meters and kilometers are much too long.

29. A: The circumference is the distance around the infant's head, i.e. the size of the infant's head. A tape measure is the only tool in the list that can measure circumference. The scale measures weight, the thermometer measures temperature, and the stethoscope is used to listen to the heartbeat.

30. C: The entire length of the figure is 16 cm and the figure has 4 segments. Therefore, each segment is 4 cm long.
$$16 \text{ cm} \div 4 = 4 \text{ cm}$$
Two segments are between segments 1 and 3. Therefore,
$$(2)(4 \text{ cm}) = 8 \text{ cm}$$

31. C: To find each percentage, divide the first number by the second number, then multiply by 100. So the percentage in answer A is $\left(\frac{50}{250}\right) \times 100 = 20$, the percentage in answer B is $\left(\frac{57}{250}\right) \times 100 = 22.8$, the percentage in answer C is $\left[\frac{(74+55)}{433}\right] \times 100 = \left(\frac{129}{433}\right) \times 100 = 29.8$, the percentage in answer D is $\left(\frac{21}{183}\right) \times 100 = 11.5$, and the percentage in answer E is $\left(\frac{5}{183}\right) \times 100 = 2.7$.

32. B: There are 37 Caucasian staff members in City Y. If we subtract this from the number of employees with 5-10 years of service in City Y (41), we see that 4 of those staff members must be non-Caucasian.

33 B: The percentage of female staff members in City Y is $\left(\frac{90}{183}\right) \times 100 = 49.2$. In City X, it is $\left(\frac{97}{250}\right) \times 100 = 38.8$. Subtracting, we see that the difference between these percentages is approximately 10.

34. B: The percentage of staff members with zero complaints in City X is $\left(\frac{202}{250}\right) \times 100 = 80.8$. In City Y, the percentage is $\left(\frac{161}{183}\right) \times 100 = 88.0$.

Science Answer Explanations

1. A: The circulatory system circulates materials throughout the entire body. The heart, blood, and blood vessels are part of the circulatory system. The kidneys, however, are part of the urinary system.

2. D: The digestive system helps the body process food and the stomach is the only item in the list that helps the body with digestive functions. The spine is part of the skeletal system, the brain is part of the nervous system, and the lungs are part of the respiratory system.

3. B: The nervous system is the center of communication for the body. The respiratory system helps the body breathe. The digestive system helps break down food, and the circulatory system carries vital materials to all the areas of the body.

4. C: The respiratory system uses the lungs, diaphragm, trachea, and bronchi to help the body breathe. The circulatory system carries blood. Food is broken down by the digestive system, and the central nervous system sends messages throughout the body.

5. D: The immune system helps the body avoid, detect, and eliminate infections. A healthy immune system should not, however, create infections.

6. B: The human body has 5 types of bone. The spine and hips are irregular bones because they do not fit the other major bone types, which are long, short, flat, and sesamoid. Choice A, curvy bones, does not describe one of the major bone types.

7. C: Most bones in the limbs are long bones, including the thighs, forearms, and fingers. The ankles, however, are not long bones because they do not have a shaft that is longer than it is wide.

8. A: Education does not directly influence the population of the United States since education does not determine how many people live in the country. Immigration, births, and deaths directly affect the number of people in the United States at any point in time.

9. D: Birth rates within a given population are influenced by the age, health, and fertility of the women within that population. In order for the population to have high birth rates, the women must be healthy, fertile, and of child bearing age.

10. D: If scientists find a cure for cancer, those who would have died from the disease would live longer. Therefore the population would most likely increase. All the other choices would most likely cause the population to decrease or would have no direct effect.

11. B: Each time 1 person dies, 2 babies are born to take that person's place. Therefore, the population is increasing. In order for the population to decrease, more people would have to die than be born. The population is changing and therefore has not reached a steady state.

12. D: The process of natural selection describes how animals survive by adapting to their environment. The animals that survive produce offspring who have the same advantageous traits and survival skills. Conversely, animals that lack such traits and skills do not live to produce offspring that may also lack them. In this case, the first two scenarios present fast zebras and polar bears with thick coats. In both cases, these animals possess traits that allow them to survive and reproduce. The third choice demonstrates how natural selection eliminates animals that lack the advantageous trait of sight.

13. B: The choices list four categories of the biological classification system. Within these four choices, the kingdom is the broadest category and the phylum is a bit more specific. The genus narrows down the classification even further, and the species is the narrowest of all the major categories.

14. A: The nucleus is the control center for the cell. The cell membrane surrounds the cell and separates the cell from its environment. Cytoplasm is the thick fluid within the cell membrane that surrounds the nucleus and contains organelles. Mitochondria are often called the power house of the cell because they provide energy for the cell to function.

15. A: Cilia and flagella are responsible for cell movement. Ribosomes are organelles that help synthesize proteins within the cell. The cell membrane helps the cell maintain its shape and protects it from the environment. Lysosomes have digestive enzymes.

16. C: Cellular differentiation is the process by which simple, less specialized cells become highly specialized, complex cells. For example, humans are multicellular organisms who undergo cell differentiation numerous times. Cells begin as simple zygotes after fertilization and then differentiate to form a myriad of complex tissues and systems before birth.

17. D: Meiosis produces cells that are genetically different, having half the number of chromosomes of the parent cells. Mitosis produces cells that are genetically identical; daughter cells have the exact same number of chromosomes as parent cells. Mitosis is useful for repairing the body while meiosis is useful for sexual reproduction.

18. B: Photosynthesis describes the process plants use to generate food from sunlight, carbon dioxide, and water. Oxygen is given off as a byproduct of photosynthesis. Animals and plants use respiration to take oxygen into the body, and carbon dioxide is a waste product of respiration.

19. C: The structure of RNA is a single helix containing 4 nucleotides. DNA, on the other hand, is a double helix containing 4 nucleotides.

20. A: The germ cell is an embryonic cell that can develop into a gamete. Therefore, only mutations in the germ cells or the gametes themselves can change an organism's offspring.

21. D: After cell division, the daughter cells should be exact copies of the parent cells. Therefore, the DNA should replicate, or make an exact copy of itself. RNA primes DNA replication.

22. A: Genes store hereditary information and thus allow hereditary traits to be passed from parents to offspring. Genes do not prohibit hereditary transmission, and genes are not known to enable any type of environmental factors.

23. C: A chromosome is a single piece of DNA that contains many genes. Genes do not, therefore, contain many chromosomes. Furthermore, the DNA double helix contains four nucleotides, not four genes.

24. B: The phenotype describes a person's observable characteristics. The genotype describes a person's genetic makeup. Environmental factors and various phenomena are not part of the phenotype.

25. D: The complete Punnett square is shown below.

	T	S
R	TR	SR
B	TB	SB

Possibility 1 corresponds to a person with the *TR* gene combination, which means the person is tall with red hair.

26. D: Refer to the complete Punnett square in the explanation for question 25. Possibility 4 corresponds to the *SB* pair of genes, which is short with black hair.

27. C: The sun is a major external source of both light and heat for Earth. Also, the sun's energy can be used for solar power. The moon only reflects the light of the sun and is not a major light source for Earth.

28. B: Oxidation refers to losing electrons, and reduction refers to gaining electrons. The two reactions always occur in pairs. In this case, the best example of a redox reaction is copper losing 2 electrons and silver gaining 2 electrons.

29. A: A catalyst increases the rate of a chemical reaction without becoming part of the reaction. Therefore, the chemist should add a catalyst. Adding an acid, base, or neutralizer may not affect the reaction rate.

30. D: Enzymes are protein molecules that serve as catalysts for certain biological reactions. Enzymes are not acids or lipids. Enzymes are definitely relevant for living organisms and do not suppress reactions.

31. C: The substance is an acid because the pH is less than 7. Pure water has a pH near 7, and bases have a pH above 7. Carcinogens cause cancer which cannot be gauged by a pH test.

32. D: A covalent bond is one in which atoms share valence electrons. Within a water molecule, one oxygen atom and two hydrogen atoms share valence electrons to yield the H_2O structure.

33. B: A water molecule contains 2 hydrogen atoms and 1 oxygen atom. Therefore the chemical formula for water is H_2O. Also, the pH of water is 7.

34. A: Potential energy is energy that is stored due to an object's position. In this case, the golf club has the most potential energy when it is highest off the ground at step 1. The potential energy is released and becomes kinetic energy in step 2. Then energy is transferred from the club to the ball in step 3.

35. C: The atomic mass of an atom is approximately equal to the number of protons plus the number of neutrons. The weight of the electrons has little effect on the overall atomic mass.

36. B: The three major components of an atom are protons, neutrons, and electrons. Protons and neutrons have positive and neutral charges while electrons are negatively charged. Protons and neutrons reside in the atomic nucleus and make up the vast majority of the atomic weight. Electrons orbit the atomic nucleus and their mass is negligible.

37. D: Ionic bonds are formed when electrons are transferred between atoms. For instance, the sodium and chlorine atoms in salt have ionic bonds because electrons are transferred from sodium to chlorine.

38. C: The atomic weight tells the mass of the element. In the table, B is the lightest element, weighing 11 atomic mass units, and O is the heaviest element, weighing 16 atomic mass units.

39. A: Both gases and liquids are free flowing with no defined shape. Therefore, both gases and liquids take on the shape of their container.

40. A: Condensation is the process of changing from a gas to a liquid. For instance, gaseous water molecules in the air condense to form liquid rain drops. Vaporization describes changing from liquid to gas. Melting is the process of changing from solid to liquid and sublimation describes changing from solid to gas.

41. D: The researcher wants to correlate smoking with premature aging. Therefore, she needs to know if the survey participants smoke. If the participant does not smoke, the data may not be relevant to the research study.

42. B: Establishing a secure Internet site could help match adopted children with the biological families and still protect everyone's privacy. The other methods are impractical and would not provide privacy protection.

43. B: The evidence says that every child in a certain family suffers from autism. All of these children have genetic commonalities. Therefore, autism may be genetic. The evidence does not mention whether the children died from autism. Therefore, no conclusion can be drawn that autism is lethal. Furthermore, nothing about the evidence leads to a conclusion that autism is "wonderful".

44. D: Decreased mortality during childbirth could be explained by any or all of the statements presented. Safer cesarean sections, health monitoring tools, and hand washing could all improve a woman's chances of surviving childbirth.

45. A: A scientific argument should discuss outcomes that are objective and measureable, such as blood pressure, energy level, and overall health. The other choices present arguments that are subjective and based on emotions instead of facts.

46. C: Conducting this investigation may reveal a group of people who need higher quality medical care. Asking wealthy people for money does not help the researcher learn more about their quality of medical care. Although helping healthy people to stay healthy is important, helping those with poor medical care is more critical.

47. B: Mathematics is inherently objective. Therefore, mathematics allows researchers to take an objective approach to analyzing their data. Scientific research does not typically include data analysis that is emotional, unrealistic, or artistic.

48. B: Fabricating research results is not a reason to include technology. Accessing large amounts of data, analyzing data, and conducting a variety of experiments are all ways that technology can benefit scientific research.

49. A: A limiting reactant is entirely used up by the chemical reaction. Limiting reactants control the extent of the reaction and determine the quantity of the product. A reducing agent is a substance that reduces the amount of another substance by losing electrons. A reagent is any substance used in a chemical reaction. Some of the most common reagents in the laboratory are sodium hydroxide and hydrochloric acid. The behavior and properties of these substances are known, so they can be effectively used to produce predictable reactions in an experiment.

50. B: The horizontal rows of the periodic table are called periods. The vertical columns of the periodic table are known as groups or families. All of the elements in a group have similar properties. The relationships between the elements in each period are similar as you move from left to right. The periodic table was developed by Dmitri Mendeleev to organize the known elements according to their similarities. New elements can be added to the periodic table without necessitating a redesign.

51. C: The mass of 7.35 mol water is 132 grams. You should be able to find the mass of various chemical compounds when you are given the number of mols. The information required to perform this function is included on the periodic table. To solve this problem, find the molecular mass of water by finding the respective weights of hydrogen and oxygen. Remember that water contains two hydrogen molecules and one oxygen molecule. The molecular mass of hydrogen is roughly 1, and the molecular mass of oxygen is roughly 16. A molecule of water, then, has approximately 18 grams of mass. Multiply this by 7.35 mol, and you will obtain the answer 132.3, which is closest to answer choice c.

52. B: 119°K is equivalent to –154 degrees Celsius. It is likely that you will have to perform at least one temperature conversion on the exam. To convert degrees Kelvin to degrees Celsius, simply subtract 273. To convert degrees Celsius to degrees Kelvin, simply add 273. To convert degrees Kelvin into degrees Fahrenheit, multiply by $\frac{9}{5}$ and subtract 460. To convert degrees Fahrenheit to degrees Kelvin, add 460 and then multiply by $\frac{5}{9}$. To convert degrees Celsius to degrees Fahrenheit, multiply by $\frac{9}{5}$ and then add 32. To convert degrees Fahrenheit to degrees Celsius, subtract 32 and then multiply by $\frac{5}{9}$.

53. A: There are four different types of tissue in the human body: epithelial, connective, muscle, and nerve. *Epithelial* tissue lines the internal and external surfaces of the body. It is like a sheet, consisting of squamous, cuboidal, and columnar cells. They can expand and contract, like on the inner lining of the bladder. *Connective* tissue provides the structure of the body, as well as the links between various body parts. Tendons, ligaments, cartilage, and bone are all examples of connective tissue. *Muscle* tissue is composed of tiny fibers, which contract to move the skeleton. There are three types of muscle tissue: smooth, cardiac, and skeletal. *Nerve* tissue makes up the nervous system; it is composed of nerve cells, nerve fibers, neuroglia, and dendrites.

54. B: The epidermis is the outermost layer of skin. The thickness of this layer of skin varies over different parts of the body. For instance, the epidermis on the eyelids is very thin, while the epidermis over the soles of the feet is much thicker. The dermis lies directly beneath the epidermis. It is composed of collagen, elastic tissue, and reticular fibers. Beneath the dermis lies the subcutaneous tissue, which consists of fat, blood vessels, and nerves. The subcutaneous tissue contributes to the regulation of body temperature. The hypodermis is the layer of cells underneath the dermis; it is generally considered to be a part of the subcutaneous tissue.

English and Language Usage Answer Explanations

1. B: Ellipses are frequently used in quotations to indicate that material has been excluded. This is certainly the case in the quoted passage in question 1. A brief section from the Declaration of Independence has been removed from the quote, and this exclusion is indicated by the ellipses. Ellipses do not indicate emphasis; they indicate that something is not included. Quotation marks indicate quoted material. Ellipses, while often used in quoted material, are not exclusive to, nor do they indicate, quoted material. Ellipses may be used regardless of the point of view, so they do not indicate a single point of view or more than one point of view.

2. C: The soldier would have received a *medal* for his display of courage, strength, and *mettle*, which is a slightly archaic (but still relevant) word that suggests bravery in the face of danger. The other answer choices contain one or more incorrect words.

3. C: The word *each* is singular, and this quality is emphasized by the singular *student*. As a result, the accompanying pronoun should be the singular *his or her*. If spoken, this sentence might contain the plural *their*, which would be more common for speech patterns. But, this is certainly not correct, and should not be used in writing. The singular *his* by itself is considered inappropriate and exclusive, and would only be correct if the context of the sentence indicated a class full of male students (which it does not). The word *ones* reads awkwardly in the sentence, and does more to confuse its meaning than to add to it.

4. D: The context suggests that Thomas Macaulay thought that people seldom apply wise sayings to avoid foolishness. The plural word in the sentence suggests the need for a plural synonym, so *advice* does not work. The word *preferences* does not make much sense in the sentence. While the statement itself is a quote – and wise sayings are usually quoted – the word *quotes* is not a synonym for *apothegms*, and is therefore not the best choice.

5. A: The word *piqued* is the correct choice, and is used to describe a heightened interest in something. The word *peaked* would be appropriate to describe height or the highest reach (e.g., his blood pressure *peaked*, and then came back down). The word *peke* is frequently used to describe a Pekingese breed of dog; therefore, *peked* does not make sense in the context of this sentence. The word *peeked* would suggest someone looking around the corner to see something.

6. A: Answer choice A includes all of the correct elements of punctuation needed to make this sentence clear and readable. In particular, there is a colon after the phrase "the following items for his class"; this indicates that a series of items will be listed. As these items do not contain internal commas, they may be separated by commas, so the rest of the punctuation in answer choice A is correct. Answer choice B uses a comma instead of a colon in front of the introductory phrase, making the series of items difficult to distinguish. Answer choice C uses semicolons instead of commas between the items in the series. The semicolons are not necessary, and make the sentence more confusing to read instead of clearer. Answer choice D uses a dash, which is not a correct way to introduce a series of items.

7. C: Answer choice C combines all of the information in the passage into a single coherent sentence. Answer choice A inexplicably states that the French and Indian War did not occur in North America, but the passage does not indicate this. Instead, the passage notes that the French and Indian War was not an isolated conflict, that it *did* occur in North America, and that it was also part of the larger Seven Years' War Europe was fighting. Answer choice B contains correct information, but is choppy rather than fluid and coherent. Answer choice B is concise, but it lacks the style and clarity of answer choice C. Answer choice D contains correct information, but it fails to explain – as stated in the original passage – that the French and Indian War was actually part of the larger Seven Years' War. Answer choice D implies that the French and Indian War was unrelated to the Seven Years' War, which contradicts the passage.

8. A: Of the answer choices, the only word that functions as a verb is *fought*. The word *control* is a noun in this sentence. The word *trade* functions either as an adjective to modify *routes*, or as a part of the single noun phrase *trade routes*. The word *those* functions as an adjective.

9. A: Only answer choice A is a simple sentence. It contains an opening phrase, but as this is a phrase instead of a dependent clause, the sentence is simple. Answer choices B and D contain a dependent clause, which makes these sentences complex. Answer choice C contains two independent clauses, which make the sentence compound.

10. C: In answer choice C, the word *empress* does not need to be capitalized, because it is not being used as a title. Instead, it is simply a description of Maria Theresa's role as empress over Austria. Answer choice A incorrectly capitalizes the word *family* twice. Answer choice B fails to capitalize the word *empire* in *Holy Roman Empire*. Answer choice D incorrectly capitalizes *province*, which is not being used as a proper noun in the sentence.

11. C: Answer choice C correctly uses double quotation marks and places the period within the quotation marks. Answer choice A uses single quotation marks. Answer choice B uses single quotation marks, and incorrectly places the period outside the quotation marks. Answer choice D correctly uses double quotation marks, but incorrectly places the period outside of them.

12. D: As the herd is apparently moving in unison across the highway, the collective noun *herd* is singular, and thus takes a singular verb. (If, however, the moose were stampeding at random, each moose in a different direction, the collective noun *herd* would be considered plural.) In answer choice A, the pronoun *some* can be either singular or plural, depending on the prepositional phrase that follows it. Because the phrase contains the singular *fervor*, the sentence needs a singular verb. (On the other hand, the phrase *some of the people* would require a plural verb, because of the plural *people*.) In answer choice B, *Gary* is the primary subject, and requires a singular verb, regardless of the phrase *as well as his three children* that sits between Gary and the verb. In answer choice C, the opening verb in this interrogative sentence is determined by whether the noun following the pronoun *neither* is singular or plural. In this case, the singular *Robert* requires that the opening verb be *is*. Note that if the order were reversed, the sentence would be correct with *are*: *Are neither his parents nor Robert planning to see the presentation*? This is fairly awkward, though, so the other form would be more common.

13. B: The word *earlier* is an adverb that modifies the verb *tried* and answers the adverb question *when*? The word *call* is part of the infinitive (i.e. noun) phrase *to call*. The word *could* is a helping verb that accompanies the verb *get*. The word *phone* functions as a noun in this sentence.

14. D: In question 14, the parenthetical statement includes information that is useful – in this case the years of Franz Joseph I's reign – but does not fit into the flow of the sentence. The writer has chosen to include the years of Franz Joseph I's reign in parentheses, instead of using a dependent clause along the lines of "...the reign of Franz Joseph I, who ruled from 1848 to 1916." The parentheses provide information that the reader would likely want to know without interrupting the flow of the sentence. There is nothing about the parenthetical remark to indicate that the numbers refer to the pages of a book; instead, the numbers make much more sense as dates. The information in answer choice B is essentially implied; if the empire collapsed after his reign, it is safe to say that 1916 marks the date of its collapse. But, this is not really the purpose of the parentheses. The purpose is to offset useful information without interrupting the flow of the sentence. It is likely that all of the information in the sentence came from one source, so the parentheses do not indicate outside material in this case.

15. A: In answer choice A, the subjective case pronoun *who* (rather than *whom*) correctly follows *person*. Additionally, the singular subject *person* is accompanied by the singular verb *needs*. In answer choice B, *nobody* is singular, and needs the singular *his or her* to follow it instead of *their*. In answer choice C, the use of *his* suggests that *every new instructor* is male. As there is nothing in the sentence to indicate this, the use of *his or her* would be more appropriate. In answer choice D, however, the use of *his or her* is not correct because of the structure of the sentence. The mention of the plural *Simeon and Ruth* makes the plural *their* correct.

16. C: Answer choice C correctly identifies that *I* is the first person and *you* is the second person. The order is also correct. The other answer choices either include an incorrect point of view or place the points of view in incorrect order.

17. B: The word *definitely* is often spelled incorrectly. (It does not help that the Spell Check option of word processing programs often overwrites any misspellings with *defiantly*.) Only answer choice B demonstrates the correct spelling. The other answer choices are either spelled incorrectly or, in the case of *defiantly*, simply indicate the wrong word.

18. A: In the sentence provided, the word *walking* is a gerund (which functions as a noun) and the subject. In this sentence, the word *walking* is not being used as an adverb, an adjective, or a conjunction. Its use as an adverb in any context would be fairly unlikely; its use as a conjunction would be virtually impossible.

19. D: The use of *malediction* in the sentence, combined with the obvious wrath of the fairy who was not invited to the princess's christening, would suggest that what the fairy utters is a *curse*. No doubt some *enchantment* is involved, but this particular word does not capture the sense of impending evil that is implied. A *remedy* will be needed to counter the effects of the curse, but this is clearly not the meaning of *malediction*. It is logical that the *malediction* is also a promise of evil to come, but the word *promise* fails to capture the negativity that is implied.

20. C: Only answer choice C combines the sentences in such a way as to maintain the original meaning of the passage, while also illustrating style and clarity. Answer choice A combines some of the information from the passage, but leaves most of it untouched. Answer choice B contains good information, but it also tweaks the original passage to suggest ideas that are not necessarily there. The original claims that Perrault's version is *one of the most familiar*. Answer choice B claims that it is *the* most familiar. The final sentence in answer choice B adds in details about the Brothers Grimm having provided their own version of the story. But, the original passage indicates that the fairy tale we know today contains elements from Perrault as well as the Brothers Grimm. Answer choice B fails to indicate this clearly. Answer choice D reverses the order of the information in the passage, but to little effect. If anything, answer choice D appears to be more about Perrault and the Brothers Grimm than about the origins of *Sleeping Beauty*. As this is not the main topic of the passage, choice D is not an effective revision.

21. D: Answer choice D correctly uses an apostrophe to indicate the possessive element within the sentence. Answer choice A incorrectly changes the plural word *fairies* into the possessive word *fairy's*. Similarly, answer choice B makes the plural *historians* possessive, and answer choice C makes the plural *seasons* possessive by changing it to the singular possessive *season's*. None of these words is possessive in the context of their respective sentences, so only answer choice D is correct.

22. C: The word *you* is always second person, and it is either singular or plural depending on its context. In the sentence provided, the teacher is speaking to a class, and the class is likely to be made up of more than one person. Therefore, the *you* in the sentence is second-person plural. The other answer choices identify the wrong point of view, and answer choices A and D incorrectly identify the word as singular.

23. D: Answer choice D contains two independent clauses, so it is a compound sentence, not a simple sentence. All of the other answer choices are simple sentences.

24. A: Someone who is committed to personal grooming is likely to be *fussy*, and this is the meaning of the word *fastidious*. The word *lazy* makes little sense in the context of the sentence. No doubt some of Poirot's activities are both *old-fashioned* and *hilarious*, but neither of these words fit the context of the sentence, and thus cannot be synonyms for *fastidious*.

25. B: The sentence indicates that the connections Miss Marple makes are *seemingly extraneous*. However, the sentence also states that she uses this information to solve mysteries. This would suggest that the word *extraneous* means *irrelevant*. This sentence implies that Miss Marple's approach appears to be meaningless, but has proven to be effective. Answer choice A indicates the very opposite of what the sentence implies. Answer choice C makes little sense in the context of the sentence. Answer choice D would work but for the adverb *seemingly*; this indicates that the connections appear to be irrelevant, but are actually not. With *seemingly* in the sentence, the meaning completely changes if *useful* is added in place of *extraneous*.

26. D: This is another word that is frequently misspelled. *Rhythm* is the correct spelling. All of the other answer choices add an unnecessary *y* and add or leave out an *h*.

27. B: For the sentence to read correctly, it must be clear that someone is leaping into the saddle when the horse bolts. In its original form, the only party identified in the sentence is the horse, and s/he cannot both leap into a saddle and bolt. Answer choice B includes the mention of a second party (an unnamed *he*), who does the leaping as the horse does the bolting. Answer choice A creates an amusing picture, but it fails to make sense of the original sentence. Answer choice C is an interesting take on the sentence, but it places the action of the sentence in an odd order. It is more likely that the bolting occurred immediately after the leaping, and not the other way around, as indicated in answer choice C: (One cannot exactly leap into a saddle after the horse has already taken off.) Answer choice D is technically correct in terms of the information it provides, but it turns a single sentence into two sentences, and it incorrectly joins them with a comma splice.

28. A: The possessive pronoun *hers* is spelled without any apostrophes. Only answer choice A correctly indicates this. The other answer choices attempt to insert an apostrophe and/or an extra *s* into the word.

29. A: If an anaesthetic creates a temporary loss of feeling or sensation, and *aesthet* means "feeling," then *an-* must mean "without." Therefore, anaesthetic means "without feeling." The other prefix meanings do not create as clear a connection to the recognized meaning of the full word *anaesthetic*. To be "against feeling" makes little sense. To be "away feeling" is meaningless. To be "before feeling" would be appropriate to describe the moments before the anaesthetic wears off, but this is a qualification rather than a clear definition.

30. C: If the years leading up to the American Civil War are described as *antebellum*, and *bellum* means "war," the only possible meaning of *ante-* is "before." *Antebellum*, therefore, means "before war." The other prefixes do little to break the word down to a sensible meaning. "Again war" and "together war" are meaningless. "Good war" does nothing to explain why the pre-Civil War years were called *antebellum*, particularly when considering the atrocities of war that were soon to follow.

31. C: The phrase *she and I* makes the sentence grammatically correct. The blank needs to be filled by the subject of the sentence. The subject of a sentence or clause is the person, place, or thing that performs the verb. There are a couple of ways to determine that this sentence needs a subject. To begin with, the blank is at the beginning of the sentence, where the subject most often is found. Also, when you read the sentence, you will notice that it is unclear who went to the movies. Because you are looking for the subject, you need the nominative pronouns *she and I*.

32. C: The word *effected* is not spelled correctly in the context of this sentence. In order to answer this question, you need to know the difference between *affect* and *effect*. The former is a verb and the latter is a noun. In other words, *affect* is something that you do and *effect* is something that is. In this sentence, the speaker is describing something that the prescription medication *did*. Therefore, the appropriate word is a verb. *Effect*, however, is a noun. For this reason, instead of *effected* the author should have used the word *affected*.

33. B: The word *hear* is not spelled correctly in the context of this sentence. The speaker has mixed up the homophones *hear* and *here*. *Homophones* are words that sound the same but are spelled differently and have a different meaning. Homophones are not to be confused with *homonyms*, which are spelled the same but have a different meaning. In question 5, the author is trying to describe the place where the climate is; that is, he or she is describing the climate *here*. Unfortunately, the author uses the word *hear*, which is a verb meaning "to listen."

34. B: The word *further* is not used correctly in the context of this sentence. Here, the word *farther* would be more appropriate. The distinction between *further* and *farther* is likely to appear in at least one question on the exam. For the purposes of the examination, you just need to know that *farther* can be used to describe physical distance, while *further* cannot. In this sentence, the speaker is describing a distance to be walked, which is a physical distance. For this reason, the word *further* is incorrect.

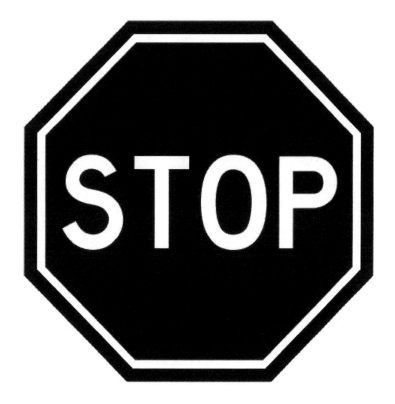

FREE Test Taking Tips DVD Offer

To help us better serve you, we have developed a Test Taking Tips DVD that we would like to give you for <u>FREE</u>. **This DVD covers world-class test taking tips that you can use to be even more successful when you are taking your test.**

All that we ask is that you email us your feedback about your study guide. Please let us know what you thought about it – whether that is good, bad or indifferent.

To get your **FREE Test Taking Tips DVD**, email <u>freedvd@studyguideteam.com</u> with "FREE Test Taking Tips DVD" in the subject line and the following information in the body of the email:

    a.   The title of your study guide.

    b.   Your product rating on a scale of 1-5, with 5 being the highest rating.

    c.   Your feedback about the study guide. What did you think of it?

    d.   Your full name and shipping address to send your free DVD.

If you have any questions or concerns, please don't hesitate to contact us at <u>freedvd@studyguideteam.com</u>.

Thanks again!

53532436R00108

Made in the USA
Lexington, KY
09 July 2016